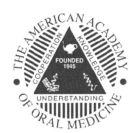

CLINICIAN'S GUIDE
Pharmacology
Dental Medicin
Second Edition

MW00837430

Editors	Contents	Pg

Jeffrey M. Casiglia, DMD, DMSc
Private Practice
Lecturer, Harvard School of Dental Medicine
Boston, Massachusetts

Peter L. Jacobsen, PhD, DDS
Adjunct Professor, Department of Pathology and
Medicine
University of the Pacific, Arthur A Dugoni School of
Dentistry
San Francisco, CA 94115

Contributing Authors

Ronald S. Brown, DDS, MS
Richard P. Cohan, AB, DDS, MS, MA, MBA, FAGD
Karen M. Crews, DMD
Michaell A. Huber, DDS
Wendy Hupp DMD
Joseph L. Konzelman, DDS
Peter B. Lockhart, DDS, MS, FDS RCSEd, FDS RCPS
Craig S. Miller, DMD, MS
Brian C. Muzyka, DMD, MS, MBA
Joel J. Napeñas, DDS, FDS RCSEd
Thomas P. Shopper, DDS, MEd
Michael A. Siegel, DDS, MS, FDS RCSEd
Nathaniel S. Treister, DMD, DMSc

Contributing authors are members of the American
Academy of Oral Medicine. This monograph represents a
consensus of the contributing authors and not
necessarily the private views of any of the individuals

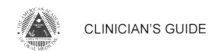
American Academy of Oral Medicine
PO Box 2016
Edmonds, WA 98020-9516
Tel: (425) 778-6162
Fax: (425) 771-9588
Email: info@aaom.com
www.Aaom.com

ISBN [print]: 978-1936176-06-9
Printed in the United States

Notice: The authors and publisher have made every effort to ensure that the patient care recommended herein, including choice of drugs and drug dosages, is in accord with the accepted standard and practice at the time of publication. However, since research and regulation constantly change clinical standards, the reader is urged to check the product information sheet included in the package of each drug, which includes recommended doses, warnings, and contraindications. This is particularly important with new or infrequently used drugs. Any treatment regimen, particularly one involving medication, involves inherent risk that must be weighed on a case-by-case basis against the benefits anticipated. The reader is cautioned that the purpose of this book is to inform and enlighten; the information contained herein is not intended as, and should not be employed as, a substitute for individual diagnosis and treatment.

The second edition of this Guide is dedicated to the memory of Jonathan A. Ship, DMD. Dr. Ship was an inspiration to a generation of students, oral medicine residents and colleagues and a revered member of the American Academy of Oral Medicine. His research contributions in geriatric dentistry, xerostomia, Sjögren's syndrome and oral, head and neck cancer will serve the professional community and society for generations. His friendship, guidance, professionalism and laughter are sorely missed by everyone who knew and loved him. Dr. Ship has contributed extensively to this Guide.

ABOUT THE AMERICAN ACADEMY OF ORAL MEDICINE (AAOM) - The AAOM is a 501c6, nonprofit organization founded in 1945 as the American Academy of Dental Medicine and took its current name in 1966. The members of the American Academy of Oral Medicine include an internationally recognized group of health care professionals and experts concerned with the oral health care of patients who have complex medical conditions, oral mucosal disorders, and / or chronic orofacial pain. Oral Medicine is the field of dentistry concerned with the oral health care of medically complex patients and with the diagnosis and non-surgical management of medically-related disorders or conditions affecting the oral and maxillofacial region.

The American Academy of Oral Medicine • (425) 778-6162 • www.aaom.com • PO Box 2016 • Edmonds • WA • 98020-9516

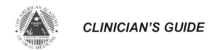
AMERICAN ACADEMY OF ORAL MEDICINE

Mission:

1. To promote the study and dissemination of knowledge of the medical aspects of dentistry while serving the best interests of the public.

2. To promote the highest standards of care in the diagnosis and treatment of oral conditions that are not responsive to conventional dental or oral maxillofacial surgical procedures.

3. To provide an avenue of referral for dental practitioners who have patients with severe, life-threatening medical disorders or complex diagnostic problems involving the oral and maxillofacial region that require ongoing nonsurgical management.

4. To improve the quality of life of patients with medically related oral disease.

5. To foster increased understanding and cooperation between medical and dental professions.

6. To obtain American Dental Association recognition of oral medicine as a specialty.

The Academy achieves these goals by holding national meetings annually; by presenting lectures, workshops, and seminars; by sponsorship of the American Board of Oral Medicine; by the editorship of the Oral Medicine Section of *OralSurgery, Oral Medicine, Oral Pathology, Oral Radiology and Endodontics*; and by publishing monographs and position papers on timely subjects relating to oral medicine.

The presented information is based on current knowledge and accepted standards of practice. Following the guidelines set forth in this monograph may not ensure successful management of every patient. This monograph represents a consensus of the editors and authors and not necessarily the private views of any individual.

All brand name medications may have patents, service marks, trademarks, or registered trademarks and are the property of their respective companies.

This *Clinician's Guide* is another AAOM educational service. Other Clinician's Guides available from the Academy include:

Treatment of Common Oral Conditions, 7/e
Tobacco Cessation 2/e
Oral Health in Geriatric Patients, 3/e
Chronic Orofacial Pain, 3/e
Medically Complex Dental Patients 4/e

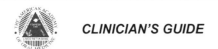
PREFACE

Thank you for the purchase of the AAOM monograph *Clinician's Guide to Pharmacology in Dental Medicine*. This publication is the culmination of a great deal of work from a wide array of authors, including a number of world leaders and widely recognized educators in their respective areas of contribution. The real challenge for us as editors has been to condense the tremendous volume of their expertise into a manageable and succinct publication without sacrificing any of the valuable information they provided. We can only hope we have succeeded in a way that does justice to the considerable time and effort they have so generously volunteered to this project.

Dentistry exists as a subspecialty of medicine. Although a significant proportion of dental treatment can be characterized as surgical in nature, pharmacologic therapy often plays an important adjunctive role in treatment. Numerous conditions exist that are not amenable to surgical intervention and can be treated only with prescribed medications. The dizzying array of conditions the dental professional may treat, combined with the ever-increasing number of available drug choices, makes it challenging to know what may be the most effective therapy. It is also difficult to remain current with what medications are available, new dosages, and new drug interactions.

It is important to mention at the outset that this publication covers a very specific range of topics. The goal of this monograph is to provide, in reasonable detail, information pertaining to the use of pharmacologic agents that may be used by the dental practitioner in general or specialty practice. The subjects are grouped by either specific classes of therapeutic agent (eg, antiviral agents) or by a pharmacologic concept (eg, reactions to pharmacologic agents). However, this volume is intended to be neither a pharmacology textbook nor a manual on the recognition and diagnosis of oral conditions. Other *Clinician's Guides* are available from the Academy of Oral Medicine that are excellent resources and specifically geared toward the diagnosis and treatment of specific oral conditions.

It is also important to note that the information provided was considered current at the time of publication, and every effort was made to ensure that it is accurate. However, the field of pharmacotherapeutics is highly dynamic; new

medications are constantly becoming available, and other agents are removed from the market if they are realized as posing a danger to consumers. Before prescribing any medication, clinicians should exercise due diligence to confirm that it is still available and that no new warnings or risks have been established since this volume's publication. To facilitate this, an entire chapter is devoted to electronic and Web-based resources that allow the practitioner to remain current and up-to-date with this ever-changing information.

Once again, thank you for the purchase of this AAOM *Clinician's Guide to Pharmacology in Dental Medicine*. We hope that it is a useful addition to your reference library and welcome suggestions for alterations and additions that may be incorporated into future editions.

Jeffrey Casiglia and Peter Jacobsen, Editors

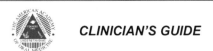
Standard Abbreviations

i	One	Prn	as needed (pro re nata)
ii	Two	Q	every
iii	Three	q2h	every 2 hours
ā	Before	q4h	every 4 hours
ac	before meals (ante cibum)	q6h	every 6 hours
ad lib	as desired (ad libitum)	q8h	every 8 hours
asap	as soon as possible	q12h	every 12 hours
AAOM	American Academy of Oral Medicine	qam	every morning
bid	twice a day (bis in die)	qd	every day (quaque die)
btl	bottle	qhs	every bedtime
c	with	qid	four times a day (quarter in die)
cap	capsule	qod	every other day
CBC	complete blood count	qpm	every evening
CDC	U. S. Center for Disease Control and Prevention	qsad	add a sufficient quantity to equal
crm	cream	qwk	every week
disp	dispense on a prescription label	RAS	recurrent aphthous stomatitis
elix	elixir	RAU	recurrent aphthous ulcer
FDA	U.S. Food and Drug Administration	RBC	red blood cell count
g	gram	RHL	recurrent herpes labialis
gtt	drop	RIH	recurrent intraoral herpes
h	hour	Rx	prescription
hs	at bedtime	ś	without
HSV	herpes simplex virus	Sig	patient dosing instructions on prescription label
IU	international units	sol	solution
IV	intravenous	SPF	sun protection factor
L	liter	stat	immediately
liq	liquid	syr	syrup
loz	lozenge	tab	tablet
mg	milligram	tbsp	tablespoon
min	minute	tid	three times a day (ter in die)
mL	milliliter	top	topical
NaF	sodium fluoride	tsp	teaspoon
oint	ointment	U	unit
OTC	over-the-counter	ut dict	as directed (ut dictum)
oz	ounce	UV	ultraviolet
p	after	visc	viscous
pc	after meals	VZV	varicella-zoster virus
PABA	para-aminobenzoic acid	WBC	white blood cell count
PHN	postherpetic neuralgia	wk	week
PLT	platlet count	yr	year
po	by mouth (per os)	Zn	zinc

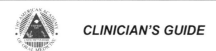
GENERAL CONSIDERATIONS FOR PHARMACOLOGIC THERAPY

The dental practitioner is responsible for a great deal of knowledge with respect to the oral cavity: knowledge of numerous disease processes, diagnosis, prevention, radiograph interpretation, and surgical and nonsurgical treatment. Although the mainstay of dental practice remains the surgical management of conditions, pharmaceutical agents often serve as important adjuncts to these procedures (eg, for control of pain and infection). However, there are also numerous conditions for which pharmacologic therapy is the only treatment indicated (eg, fungal and viral infections).

This monograph attempts to provide a reasonable overview of a wide array of pharmaceutical agents that the dental practitioner may need to prescribe. Although the scope of practice differs from clinician to clinician, an effort has been made to emphasize those medications with special relevance to and most frequently prescribed by dentists and specialists within dental medicine. The editors and authors appreciate that this publication is not a comprehensive review of all pharmacologic agents available to treat every possible condition. There are numerous other published volumes to serve this purpose. There are also many electronic references available that can be continuously updated to remain current with the ever-changing array of available medications. An entire chapter that introduces and provides information on obtaining these references is included in this publication.

Certain issues remain common to all pharmacotherapeutic agents, irrespective of their specific action, and caution should be exercised with all prescribed medications. These considerations are outlined below:

- *Review of medical history.* The actions and potential adverse reactions of any pharmaceutical agent should be carefully measured against the patient's systemic health conditions. Can the patient tolerate the medication? Will it produce effects that exacerbate systemic conditions of the patient? Is it necessary to screen the patient for any metabolic disorder that might result in dangerous conditions if the drug is prescribed?
- *Review of current medications.* Any potentially prescribed agents must be compared with the patient's current medication list. When evaluating the new drug, several questions must be considered with respect to the patient's other medications:

    - *Drug action*: Does the drug's primary action increase or enhance the action of any medication the patient is already taking? Does the action of the drug counteract any of the therapeutic effects of any of the patient's medications?
    - *Drug side effect*: Does the medication have any side effects that might exacerbate one of the patient's current medical conditions?
    - *Drug metabolism*: Does the medication alter the metabolism of any other drugs that the patient is taking? Will this result in increased or decreased levels of drugs that can produce life-threatening effects or require altered dosing of medications?

- *Review of drug allergies.* Before pharmaceutical agents can be prescribed, patients must be interviewed for previous allergic reactions to medications. Any drugs that have previously produced side effects, such as rash, swelling, or anaphylaxis, must obviously be avoided. It is also important to check for cross-reactions for drugs to which patients have allergies, such as cephalosporins in penicillin-allergic patients. Finally, drug sensitivities should be taken into consideration, although the reactions are not life threatening. Medications that have induced nausea, for example, on previous

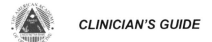
administration should be avoided and another agent substituted if at all possible. Similarly, epinephrine might be avoided in patients who complain of being "jittery" after anesthesia administration.

- *Review of systems.* A patient's medical and drug histories are important. However, the review of systems, whereby the patient is questioned with respect to their current symptoms, is invaluable in possibly realizing occult medical conditions and pathology. Depending on what symptoms, if any, are realized during the review of systems, the choice of medication prescribed may be delayed or altered. For example, if a patient reveals that he or she has been experiencing fatigue and lethargy, this may change the decision to prescribe a medication that has the side effect of sedation or another drug that may produce anemia. The review of systems may also reveal circumstances that necessitate referral to the patient's physician prior to the initiation of pharmacotherapy.

- *Other interactions.* Are there other substances with which the drug may interact or that may impact the metabolism or efficacy of the agent? Is it necessary for the patient to avoid certain foods while taking the drug? Is it important that the patient take the drug with certain foods to increase its absorption? Does the patient need to avoid other environmental exposures, such as sunlight?

- *Potential for abuse.* Does the drug in question have the potential for abuse or dependency? Does the patient have a history of substance abuse or dependency on a similar medication, alcohol, or other illicit drugs? If the patient requires narcotic analgesics, is the individual's complaint objectively verifiable, or is there the possibility that the patient is specifically seeking drugs? If this appears to be the case, conversations with the patient's family or other health care providers may be warranted.

- *Drug monitoring.* If the drug is prescribed to treat a chronic condition or the patient will be taking the drug for a prolonged period, how is the patient to be monitored? How often should the patient be seen to evaluate the response to the medication? Does the drug require periodic dose escalation to achieve therapeutic effect? Does the agent require titration to reduced levels once the effect has been realized? Does the drug require periodic monitoring of serum levels? Does the drug impact hematologic values or other serum chemistry, making it necessary to send the patient for laboratory values at regular intervals? Finally, if the medication is used for an extended period of time before being discontinued, does the possibility of withdrawal or other systemic consequence exist that necessitates the agent be tapered until therapy is complete?

These considerations should be reviewed for any drug prescribed to a patient. If it is the clinician's first time using the pharmacologic agent in question, these parameters serve as reasonable guidelines that should help in the decision-making process. However, there is no substitute for reading the manufacturer's package insert information and understanding a drug's mechanism of action, indications, contraindications, and possible side effects. Finally, if there any questions about an agent's possible systemic impact, the patient's physician should be consulted.

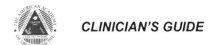
1 – TREATMENT OF BACTERIAL INFECTIONS

Bacterial infections in the oral cavity manifest as an abscess or cellulitis. An abscess occurs when the organisms, and the white cells that the body has mobilized to fight them, have focused in one location. A fluid containing this cluster of organisms and white cells is called pus. Cellulitis is characterized by swelling and redness with no obvious focus or localization of organisms - it is primarily the body's inflammatory response to the presence of infection. Different organisms have different propensities to cause either cellulitis or abscesses.

RATIONALE

An antibiotic is needed if the infection appears to be spreading or causing systemic problems such as fever or malaise (Tables 1- 1 and 1 - 2). They must also be considered if the patient has medical problems including immunosuppression (e.g., long-term steroid treatment) or systemic conditions that can impair the body's ability to fight infection (e.g., diabetes mellitus).

TREATMENT

The primary function of antibiotics is to control infection by either preventing organisms from multiplying (bacteriostatic) or killing them (bacteriocidal). The body's immune system destroys whatever is left. Proper incision and drainage is an important aspect of eliminating bacterial organisms that is often overlooked. The greater the swelling and bulk of organisms, the more important it becomes to establish drainage.

It may be useful to start the patient with a *loading dose* of the antibiotic. In these circumstances, the first dose of the drug is doubled. This increases the serum levels rapidly and more quickly achieves therapeutic serum levels of the drug.

The primary drugs of choice for odontogenic infections are penicillin or amoxicillin.

If the infection has been present for 48 to 72 hours, or if there is no response in 48 to 72 hours:

1. Clindamycin (best choice) *or*
2. Erythromycin or azithromycin *or*
3. Some dentists elect to add metronidazole to the penicillin family drug, rather than switch to clindamycin or azythromycin.

If there is no response to the azithromycin/erythromycin or the addition of metronidazole to the penicillin drug within 24 to 48 hours, then use clindamycin. Incision and drainage should be accomplished, if possible and appropriate.

Caution: All antibiotics, especially clindamycin, carry the risk of pseudomembranous colitis, which is an overgrowth of the organism *Clostridium difficile*, and manifests as watery diarrhea, cramping, and sometimes fever. If any allergy or unexpected reaction occurs, patients should immediately discontinue the medication and contact the prescriber or their primary care physician.

ALLERGY

If patient is allergic to penicillin, the first drug of choice is clindamycin.

If there is no response in 48 to 72 hours, switch to azythromycin. Erythromycin is no longer the drug of choice if a patient has a penicillin allergy. Erythromycin has too many side effects and is associated with too many drug-drug interactions.

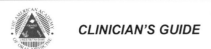
TABLE 1 - 1: SUMMARY OF DRUGS OFCHOICE TO TREAT BACTERIAL INFECTIONS

Drug (Trade Name)	Dose	No. of Tablets (7-Day Course)	Dosing Frequency
Penicillin family drugs			
Penicillin VK (Pen Vee K)	500 mg	28	qid
Amoxicillin (Trimox)	500 mg	21	tid
Amoxicillin (Trimox)	875 mg	14	bid
Cephalexin* (Keflex)	500 mg	28	Qid
Penicillins with anti-penicillinase activity			
Dicloxacillin† (Dycill)	500 mg	28	Qid
Augmentin‡	500/125 mg	21	Tid
Augmentin‡	875/125 mg	14	Bid
Macrolide antibiotics			
Erythromycin§ (E-Mycin)	250 mg	28	Qid
Clarithromycin (Biaxin)	500 mg	14	Bid
Other antibiotics useful in penicillin -allergic patients			
Clindamycin‖ (Cleocin)	300 mg	28	Qid
Azithromycin# (Zithromax)	250 mg	6	Qid
Metronidazole** (Flagyl)	500 mg	21	Tid

* Fifteen percent of patients allergic to peniciilin will also have allergies to cephalexin.

† Dicloxacillin has anti–β-lactamase activity.

‡ Augmentin contains clavulanic acid (potassium clavulanate), which is the anti-β-lactamase component of the drug. It is the second number listed (125 mg/pill).

§ Macrolides exhibit potent interactions with the liver's P450 enzyme system, prolonging the action or duration of other drugs. This can lead to potentially life-threatening reactions, and the patient's other medications should be carefully reviewed. This effect is significant for clarithromycin and erythromycin, but not azithromycin.

‖ Clindamycin may cause pseudomembranous colitis more frequently than other antibiotics.

Azithromycin comes in a "Z-Pack." Two pills are taken the first day, then one pill for 5 days.

* Metronidazole is most often prescribed in conjunction with penicillin/amoxicillin to increase the former's spectrum. Patients must avoid consuming alcohol during and for up to 3 days after taking this medication.

TABLE 1 - 2: PEDIATRIC DOSING

Drug	(mg/kg)	Dosing Frequency	Maximum Pediatric Dose (mg/kg) (Daily)
Penicillin	8–33	tid	25 – 100
Dicloxacillin	6–25	qid	25 – 100
Azithromycin	20–25	qid	75 – 100
Metronidazole	20–25	qid	75 – 100
Clindamycin	3–8	tid	10 – 25

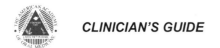

2 – Management of Oral Viral Infections

Viral infections are common occurrences in the oral cavity. Infections occur at all ages and as lytic, latent, or persistent infections. Lytic infections (e.g., human herpesviruses, coxsackievirus) often produce acute symptoms and oral mucosal ulcerations. In contrast, latent and persistent infections (herpesvirus and human papillomavirus infections) can result in episodic ulcerations and benign epithelial growths and/or induce premalignant and malignant transformation. The primary viruses of concern to dentists are the human herpesviruses (HHVs). This family of deoxyribonucleic acid (DNA) viruses includes the herpes simplex viruses (HSV-1 and HSV-2), varicella-zoster virus (VZV or HHV-3), Epstein-Barr virus (HHV-4), cytomegalovirus (HHV-5), the lymphotrophic viruses (HHV-6 and HHV-7), and Kaposi's sarcoma–associated herpesvirus (HHV-8).

A number of drugs have been formally licensed and are widely used for their specific antiviral effects (Table 2-1).Most antiviral agents specific for oral infections interrupt the lytic cycle by inhibiting replication of the virus genetic material (DNA or ribonucleic acid). The nucleoside analogs are highly selective because the herpesvirus- (HSV and VZV) specific thymidine kinase is in much greater abundance in virus-infected cells compared with uninfected cells.

HSV-1 and HSV-2 are the most common viruses in the oral cavity. HSV-1 infects 70% of the population and produces symptomatic recurrent lesions in 25% of those infected. Recurrent infections occur after stress or trauma and typically present as painful vesicles and ulcers of the lips, attached gingiva, and palate. Treatment of primary HSV-1 infection, in otherwise healthy patients, requires the use of topical and systemic analgesics and antiviral agents. Dyclonine, viscous lidocaine, Benadryl Elixir, and Benadryl with Kaopectate are effective topical anesthetics when used as a rinse for 2 minutes every 2 hours. Antiviral drugs are most effective if used early in the course of the infection (first 2 days) and are provided systemically. Topical antiviral drugs do not penetrate well and are generally recommended for recurrent episodes. Antiviral agents are beneficial when used prophylactically and intermittently by those suffering from frequent and predictable recurrences.

BELL'S PALSY

Bell's palsy is a condition caused by inflammation or trauma to the facial (cranial) nerve (VII). It is characterized by acute, unilateral, peripheral facial paresis, facial muscle weakness, and altered taste. One in 60 people are affected during their lifetime. The main causative agent is HSV-1. Other causes include facial trauma, infections with VZV, Borrelia burgdorferi (Lyme disease), human immunodeficiency virus (HIV), and tumors of the central nervous system. For viral-induced Bell's palsy, recommended therapy includes combining the anti-inflammatory properties of corticosteroids (i.e., prednisone) with an antiviral drug. About 70% of patients recover completely. However, early interceptive treatment improves the chances of full recovery by 20% and reduces the risk of postherpetic neuralgia.

VARICELLA-ZOSTER VIRUS

Varicella (chickenpox) is a highly contagious systemic infection characterized by fever and a widespread rash. The macular skin lesions turn into vesicles, and are infrequently observed in the oral cavity. Lesions resolve as patient antibody titers rise and control the infection. The virus then remains latent in sensory ganglionic neurons. Reactivation of VZV (shingles) occurs in 20% of the infected population. The likelihood of shingles increases with each passing decade. Shingles produces vesicles and pustules that extend to and abruptly stop at the midline. At cutaneous sites, the lesions eventually crust over. The risk of chickenpox and shingles is greatly reduced by administration of the live-attenuated vaccine (Varivax). The vaccine is currently recommended for infants, and a modified version (Zostavax) is recommended for adults 60 years and older. Antiviral agents are recommended for the treatment of the primary infection in persons who are more likely to develop serious disease, including persons with chronic skin or lung disease, otherwise healthy individuals 13 years of age or older, and persons receiving steroid therapy. Treatment of shingles involves antiviral drugs administered early in the outbreak generally for one week or for as long as new lesions are developing. Corticosteroids (prednisone, 60 mg/d), used in combination, improve patient quality of life and are tapered in dose over 10 to 14 days. Steroids should not be used in patients with significant hypertension, osteoporosis, diabetes mellitus or malignancy.

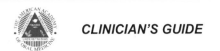
TABLE 2 - 1: DRUGS OF CHOICE TO TREAT HERPES SIMPLEX VIRUS

Drug	Available Dose	Dosing Regimens
Antiviral medications—topical		
Acyclovir (Zovirax)	5% ointment, 15 g tube	Apply thin layer to lesions 6 x / d for 7 d
Penciclovir (Denavir)	1% ointment, 2 g tube	Apply every 2 h during waking hours for 4 d
Docosanol (Abreva)	2 g tube, available OTC	Apply to lesion 5 times per day for 4 d
Antiviral medications—systemic		

Acyclovir (Zovirax)	400 mg & 800 mg tablet	Primary HSV infection
		    800 mg 5 x / d for 7–10 d
		    400 mg 3 x / d for 7–10 d
		    800 mg 2 x / d for 7–10 d
		Recurrent HSV infection
		    400 mg 3 x / d for 5 d
		    800 mg 2 x / d for 5 d
		Suppression*
		    400 mg 2 x / d
		Treatment of varicella-zoster infection
		    800 mg 5 x / d for 7 d

Valacyclovir (Valtrex)	500 mg & 1,000 mg caplet	Primary HSV infection
		    1.0 g 2 x / d for 7 – 10 d
		Recurrent HSV infection
		    2.0 g at first sign of recurrence, then 2.0 g 12 h later
		Suppression*
		    500 – 1,000 mg once daily
		Prophylaxis due to known precipitating event
		    2.0 g twice on the day of the dental procedure or event, then 1.0 g twice the next day (up to 1 – 3 days after procedure or event)
		Treatment of varicella-zoster infection
		    1.0 g 3 x / d for 7 -14 d
		Treatment of Bell's palsy
		    1.0 g 3 x / d for 7 – 10 d and prednisone 1 mg/kg/d (40 to maximum of 80 mg) in the morning for the first week; taper by 10 mg daily over second week

Famciclovir (Famvir)	125 mg, 250 mg tablet	Primary HSV infection
		    250 mg 3 x / d for 7 – 10 d
		Recurrent HSV infection
		    125 mg 2 x / d for 5 d
		Suppression*
		    250 mg 2 x / d
		Treatment of varicella-zoster infection
		    500 mg 3 x / d for 7 -14 d

OTC = over-the-counter.
All antiviral drugs should be started at the first sign of an attack to provide optimum benefit.
*Dosage may need to be adjusted in patients with frequent recurrences and in immunosuppressed patients.

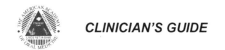
3 – TREATMENT OF FUNGAL INFECTIONS

Dentists are frequently called on to evaluate and manage oral mycotic infections. Candidosis, the most commonly occurring oral fungal infection in the nonimmunocompromised patient, is usually caused by *Candida albicans*. Up to 60% of healthy individuals harbor this fungal organism as host flora in the oral cavity. In individuals who have *Candida albicans* as a normal component of their oral microflora, their own immune system and the competing bacteria keep the fungal organisms from overgrowing. This opportunistic infection may occur owing to a variety of systemic factors or as a result of local changes in the oral environment.

Systemic conditions associated with the development of candidosis include endocrine disturbances such as diabetes, pregnancy, and hypoparathyroidism. Other systemic factors that may favor the development of candidosis include immunosuppression, as seen in patients with acquired immune deficiency syndrome (AIDS), Sjögren's or sicca syndrome, and malabsorption and malnutrition. Immunosuppression may also be iatrogenic, such as that produced by systemic steroid therapy, organ transplant anti-rejection therapy, or cancer chemotherapy. Local factors that favor the development of candidosis include changes in the oral flora resulting from decreased tissue resistance from hyposalivation, chronic local irritants (dentures, orthodontic appliances, smoking), and/or antibiotic or asthma inhaler therapy.

The clinical appearance of oral candidosis can vary greatly. Pindborg reported four clinical varieties of oral candidosis found in human immunodeficiency virus (HIV)-infected individuals: pseudomembranous, erythematous, hyperplastic, and angular cheilosis. The two most common oral presentations are pseudomembranous candidosis and erythematous candidosis (denture sore mouth). Pseudomembranous candidosis is characterized by the presence of white curd-like lesions that can be easily removed with an instrument or gauze to expose an erythematous, eroded surface underneath. Erythematous candidosis is frequently noted in patients who wear maxillary complete or partial dentures, especially in cases in which the prosthesis is not removed prior to bedtime. Clinically, erythematous candidosis appears as red, atrophic lesions. Hyperplastic candidosis is unlike the pseudomembranous and erythematous forms in that it cannot be wiped off the mucosa. Lesions of hyperplastic candidosis that do not respond to a trial of antifungal medication must be biopsied to establish a diagnosis. Finally, angular cheilosis is due to candidal infection of the labial commissures. It is characterized by redness and/or fissures radiating from one or both corners of the mouth and is often associated with small white plaques. Angular cheilosis has long been associated with vitamin B deficiency and decreased vertical dimension of occlusion. The diagnosis of candidosis can often be made from the patient's history and the clinical appearance and distribution of the mucosal lesions.When necessary, especially in an immunocompromised individual, identification of the organisms can be made from a cytology smear stained with periodic acid–Schiff reagent, a wet smear macerated with 10% potassium hydroxide, or tissue biopsy.

Oral candidosis is most often treated with topical antifungal agents such as troches or rinses (Table 3-1). Oral preparations in the form of troches provide the advantage of prolonged contact of the medication with the lesions. They are safe to use because of their poor systemic absorption. Oral hygiene must be reinforced when prescribing oral antifungal troches because they contain sucrose.The sugar content of these medications can present a problem when prescribed for diabetic patients who are on a strict carbohydrate diet or elderly patients with reduced salivary flow who are more caries prone. In these cases, it is sometimes better to substitute the vaginal preparation, which contains no sugar. Although nystatin suspension is frequently prescribed, rinses are, in general, less effective than other forms of topical antifungal therapy owing to insufficient duration of tissue contact. For rinses to be effective, they must contact the affected mucosal surfaces for a period of 3 minutes four times daily for the entire duration of therapy.

Patients who wear dentures must remove the dentures prior to using an antifungal rinse or troche unless it is treated with ointment applied to the denture itself.When treating cases of erythematous candidosis under a denture, the prosthetic appliance must be addressed, as well as the oral infection. Patients should be reminded to remove their dentures at bedtime and soak them overnight in an antifungal solution.Most commercially available denture soaking tablets are fungicidal; it should not be necessary to prescribe nystatin suspension specifically for this purpose. However, it is also possible to soak dentures

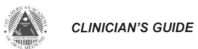 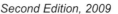

in chlorhexidine or a dilute solution of bleach (1 tsp for 8 oz of water) for the duration of antifungal therapy. The use of even a mild bleach solution for soaking dentures may affect the color of the prosthesis, and the prosthesis must be thoroughly rinsed before replacing it in the mouth.

Angular cheilosis is a mixed infection of Candida albicans and salivary species of streptococci. These lesions respond very well to combination therapy containing an antifungal and a topical steroid in a cream or ointment vehicle. Nystatin with triamcinolone acetonide or clotrimazole with betamethasone dipropionate preparations are quite useful for this purpose. Patients should be encouraged not to lick the lesions because this will serve to further superinfect the cheilosis with salivary bacteria. If the combination of medications is not readily available, the patient can be prescribed the two creams and mix a small amount of each in the palm of the hand before applying to the area.

In cases of refractory or mucocutaneous candidosis, patients in whom compliance is a problem, or women who have a concurrent candidal vaginitis, systemic antifungal therapy with ketaconazole or fluconazole is recommended. If either of these medications is used for longer than 2 weeks, liver function tests should be performed to monitor potential hepatotoxicity. A new class of antifungal medications known as echinocandins is available to treat resistant fungal infections in immunocompromised patients. These medications (caspofungin, micafungin, anidulafungin) are not currently recommended for the management of acute candidosis.

Caution: Ketaconazole and fluconazole are potent inhibitors of the hepatic microsomal enzyme system CYP3A4. As such, drug interactions must be anticipated in patients concurrently taking anticoagulant, antihistamine, antianxiety, and cholesterol-lowering medications. If patients fail to respond to systemic therapy, they should be referred to an infectious disease specialist for evaluation of resistant strains or the diagnosis must be reevaluated.

TABLE 3 – 1: SUMMARY OF DRUGS OF CHOICE TO TREAT FUNGAL INFECTIONS

Medication	Dosage	Amount	Frequency	Special Directions
Topical medications for intraoral candidosis				
Nystatin rinse	1:1,000,000 U/mL	500 mL	15 mL qid	Swish for 3 min and spit or swallow if evidence of esophageal involvement
Nystatin ointment	100,000 U/g	30 g tube	tid	Apply to inside of denture after meals
Clotrimazole troches*	10 mg	70 troches	5 x / d	Dissolve slowly in mouth. Do not chew!
Systemic treatment for candidosis				
Fluconazole†	100 mg tablets	15 tablets	qd	Take two tablets on day one
Ketoconazole†	200 mg tablets	14 tablets	qd	
Treatment for angular cheilosis				
Mycolog ointment‡	Nystatin 100,000 U/g & Triamcinolone 1%	30 g tube	qid	Apply after meals and at bedtime for 2 wk
Lotrisone‡	Clotrimazole 1% & Betamethasone 0.05%	45 g tube	qid	Apply after meals and at bedtime for 2 wk
Vytone‡	Hydrocortisone 1% & Iodoquinol 1%	28 g tube	qid	Apply after meals and at bedtime for 2 wk
Kuric‡	Ketoconazole 2%	25 g tube	qd	Apply immediately prior bedtime for 2 wk

*Consider vaginal (sugar free) preparations for patients with hyposalivation or carbohydrate-restricted diets.

†Azole systemic antifungal agents can profoundly alter the metabolism of other drugs. Caution must be exercised. Consult the patient's physician if there is any question regarding impact of antifungal therapy.

‡Patients should be advised not to lick the commissures after application of treatment

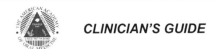

4 – MANAGEMENT OF ACUTE DENTAL PAIN

Pain is the single greatest motivator in patients seeking dental treatment that is not part of planned or routine care. In addition to this, many procedures that are performed in the dental office can produce varying levels of postoperative pain. Therefore, pain management is a critical aspect of providing quality care to patients.

In a broad sense, pharmacologic pain management can be divided into two categories: non-narcotic agents and agents with a narcotic component. The former class is composed mostly of nonsteroidal anti-inflammatory drugs (NSAIDs), whereas the latter usually consists of a narcotic agent paired with another nonnarcotic compound (so-called "combination analgesics").

NSAIDs produce analgesia principally by blocking the cyclooxygenase (COX) enzyme pathway's production of prostaglandins, yielding a reduction in inflammation and the concomitant pain response. In fact, NSAIDs are the only analgesics described herein that have a direct anti-inflammatory effect. NSAIDs are divided into nonselective (those that block the COX-1 and COX-2 isoforms) and selective (those that block COX-2 only).

The advantage of selective COX-2 inhibitors is presumably that they reduce the unwanted sequelae of gastrointestinal upset and inhibition of platelet aggregation. They are not, however, more effective in producing analgesia than nonselective agents and are much more expensive. In the months preceding publication of this document the COX-2 inhibitors have been under scrutiny for the possibility of producing adverse cardiac events. Increased risks of thrombotic events have been reported in individuals with long-term use of the agents. It does seem however, that these drugs are completely safe for consistent short-term (2 weeks or less) treatment of acute pain in individuals unable to tolerate nonselective NSAIDs.

Narcotic analgesics are usually derivatives of the opiate family and produce analgesia via stimulation of the opiate receptors. For pain management in the outpatient setting, small amounts of these agents are typically coupled with aspirin, acetaminophen, or ibuprofen for a synergistic effect, although some are available individually. The greatest concern with prescribing narcotics is in their potential for abuse, which is beyond the scope of this monograph. Practitioners should be aware of the signs of drug-seeking behavior but should not be so crippled with this fear that they fail to adequately treat pain. Opiates can also cause gastrointestinal upset, sedation, constipation, and respiratory depression. One drug included in this section, tramadol (Ultram), is a synthetic opiate agonist and is not scheduled by the Drug Enforcement Administration (DEA). However, patients can abuse the drug, develop dependence, and undergo withdrawal with abrupt discontinuation; it is therefore recommended that this agent be afforded the same respect as other "true" narcotics.

Interestingly, when contemplating dosing, the greatest consideration must be given to the non-narcotic portion of combination drugs. Because tolerance can be developed to the opiate components of combination analgesics (and owing to the comparatively small amount of opiate compared with the non-narcotic drug), the non-narcotic agent is usually the dose-limiting component. Although these drugs contain carefully regulated and abusable agents, care must be taken to remember the contraindications of the seemingly more innocuous over-the-counter components. For example, combination analgesics with aspirin and ibuprofen must be avoided in those individuals taking anticoagulants or other agents that could be displaced by aspirin's high protein-binding affinity. This can lead to dangerously high levels of other concomitantly administered drugs.

Finally, DEA scheduling can play a role in the selection of an appropriate pain management agent. The DEA ranks narcotics in order of abuse potential from II to V (there is a schedule I, but these drugs (such as cocaine) generally cannot be prescribed). Although schedule II drugs are the most potent, they are the most abusable and, hence, cannot be prescribed by telephone or prescribed with additional refills. Other medications scheduled III or higher (numerically) can be refilled or prescribed by telephone. This is an important consideration in acute pain situations when a patient may call the provider after office hours at home.

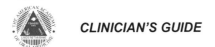

TABLE 4 - 1: DRUGS OF CHOICE FOR TREATMENT OF ACUTE PAIN

NSAIDs	Pharmacologic Agent	Side Effects
Nonselective NSAIDs	Aspirin 325 mg Ibuprofen 200, 400, 600, 800 mg Naproxen sodium 220, 275, 550 mg Ketoprofen 25, 50 mg Diflunisal 500 mg	Can cause GI upset and prolonged bleeding Contraindicated in patients with gastric ulcers, those taking anticoagulant therapy, those with established bleeding problems Indicated for mild to moderate pain
COX-2 selective	Celecoxib (Celebrex) 100, 200 mg Valdecoxib (Bextra) 10, 20 mg	Can cause GI upset and bleeding but not particularly effective for dental pain; less effective than nonselective NSAIDs

Analgesic (FDA Schedule)	Formulations Available	Trade Name	Indications
Combination Agents			
Aspirin or acetaminophen and propoxyphene (IV)	Aspirin or acetaminophen 325 mg and Propoxyphene 50 or 100 mg	Darvon-N 50, Darvocet-N 100	Mild-moderate pain
Aspirin or acetaminophen and pentazocine (IV)	Aspirin or acetaminophen 325 mg or 650 mg and Pentazocine 50 or 100 mg	Talwin, Talacet	Moderate pain
Acetaminophen with codeine (III)	Acetaminophen 325 mg and 5, 15, 30, or 60 mg codeine (Tylenol No. 1, 2, 3, and 4, respectively)	Tylenol 1 – 4	Mild to moderate pain
Ibuprofen and hydrocodone (III)	Ibuprofen 200mg and hydrocodone 7.5 mg	Vicoprofen	Moderate
Acetaminophen or aspirin and hydrocodone (III)	Aspirin 325 mg or acetaminophen 325, 500, 660 mg and Hydrocodone 5, 7.5, or 10 mg	Lortab / Lorcet, Vicodin, Norco	Moderate
Acetaminophen or aspirin and oxycodone (II)	Aspirin 325 mg or acetaminophen 325, 500, 660 mg and Oxycodone 5, 7.5, or 10 mg	Endocet, Percodan, Percocet, Roxicet, Tylox	Moderate to severe
Ibuprofen and oxycodone	Ibuprofen 400 mg and Oxycodone 5 mg	Combunox	Moderate to severe
Tramadol and acetaminophen	Acetaminophen 325 mg and Tramadol 37.5 mg	Ultracet	Mild to moderate pain
Individual agents			
Tramadol (not scheduled)	Tramadol HCl 50mg	Ultram	Mild to moderate pain
Pentazocine (IV)	Pentazocine 50 mg, Pentaozocine 50 mg and Naloxone 0.5 mg	Talwin, Pentawin, Penzyl, Tozine	Mild to moderate
Propoxyphene (IV)	Propoxyphene 65 mg	Darvon compound	Mild to moderate pain
Hydromorphone (II)	Hydromorphone 2, 4, 8 mg	Dilaudid	Severe
Meperidine (II)	Meperidine HCl 50, 100 mg	Demerol	Severe

COX-2 = cyclooxygenase-2; GI = gastrointestinal; NSAID = nonsteroidal anti-inflammatory drug.

Recommended daily maximum values for analgesic agents: ibuprofen, 2,400 mg; aspirin, 3,600 mg; acetaminophen, 4,000 mg; naproxen sodium, 1,375 mg; pentazocine, 600 mg; propoxyphene, 600 mg.

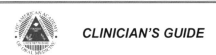
At the time of publication, the FDA was considering removal of combination analgesics from the market (and stronger regulation of acetaminophen) due to an increase in the number of reports of acetaminophen toxicity. Currently, the maximum dose is four (4) g per day, with no more than one (1) gram in a single dose. However, the FDA has voted to recommend lowering the maximum single dose to 650 mg, and has also agreed to lower the recommended maximum daily dose; though a new ceiling has not been published. Patients should be counseled not to consume combination analgesics with products such as Ny-Quil, Theraflu, or other over-the-counter remedies, as these products also contain the drug. Though safe when used at acceptable doses, acetaminophen-containing products must be used very judiciously or avoided completely in patients with advanced liver disease.

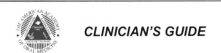
5 – Treatment of Chronic Orofacial Pain

Chronic pain is defined as "pain persisting beyond the normal healing time (usually three months) and without apparent biologic value." Treatment of chronic pain differs considerably in comparison with that of acute oral pain. Whereas drugs for acute pain typically demonstrate efficacy within minutes to hours, drugs for chronic pain often take weeks or even months to exert their effect. The pharmaceuticals used for treating acute pain are generally well understood, predictable, and effective in most individuals. In contrast, many, if not most, chronic pain therapies are nonspecific, and their efficacy varies from patient to patient. It follows from this that patients unresponsive to one therapeutic modality may benefit from another drug, possibly from the same or a different class. Put succinctly, the treatment of chronic pain, much like its origins, is complicated and frequently requires significant patience and "tweaking."

The most important aspect of treating chronic pain conditions is to first establish a definitive diagnosis. Some chronic pain conditions may be manifestations of other systemic diseases or central nervous system (CNS) dysfunction. The treating clinician must have significant knowledge of these conditions and be aware of serious etiologies that must be ruled out via advanced imaging, biopsy, laboratory studies, and collaboration with medical specialists as necessary. Most treatments for chronic orofacial pain involve altering the function of the CNS in some fashion or another. As a result of this, serious sequelae may be realized, and clinicians must be well trained to anticipate and appreciate these consequences and alter therapy appropriately.

Pain control for neuropathic pain is rated by "number needed to treat" (NNT). This number is defined as the number of patients that must be treated with the drug to find one patient who experiences greater than 50% pain relief. This functions as a rating system for efficacy comparison: the lower the NNT number, the better the efficacy.

With respect to nonspecific chronic pain, NNT values have been previously reported of 1.4 to 2.4 for tricyclic antidepressants (TCAs), 6.7 for selective serotonin reuptake inhibitors, 3.3 for carbamazepine, 1.9 for dextromethorphan, 3.7 for gabapentin, 3.4 for tramadol, and 5.9 for capsaicin.

Drugs used to treat chronic pain are borrowed from several pharmacologic categories, many of which are used in an "off-label" capacity or with doses very different from those used in the diseases they were approved to treat. These include antidepressants, anticonvulsants, benzodiazepines, and drugs from other categories (Table 5-1). Other drugs used to treat chronic pain include tramadol, which is an atypical, narcotic-like drug; dextromethorphan, which has an unknown chronic pain mechanism; and capsaicin, which down-regulates nociception. The precise mechanism by which many of the drugs used to treat chronic pain exert their effects is unknown.

The long-term use of narcotics to treat chronic pain remains a controversial subject. Although narcotics are typically used in the short term to treat acute pain, studies have demonstrated efficacy for chronic pain as well. In this situation, the drugs are typically dosed at regular intervals or provided in a time-release form or via other delivery vehicles, such as the fentanyl (Duragesic) patch. When used long term, patients develop tolerance to many of the untoward side effects that most narcotics carry. There are the real risks of physical and psychological dependence with these drugs, but they still can represent effective treatment in difficult-to-treat individuals. Use of these medications in the long term should be reserved for clinicians with significant experience in this arena.

As mentioned, many of the drugs used to treat chronic pain typically require a more specialized scope of knowledge than most general dentists have acquired. However, drugs such as TCAs have a wide safety margin and are usually manageable within a general dentistry setting. These drugs usually take 2 to 3 weeks to demonstrate any clinical benefit. Common side effects include dry mouth, drowsiness, and weight gain with prolonged use. The initial drowsiness usually subsides within the first week of use. Other side effects are also possible. After 4 weeks, if there is no perceived benefit, the dosage may be increased by one 10 to 25 mg tablet, or, if the patient can tolerate it, another dose can be added. After another month, another tablet can be added, continuing up to 75 mg. If pain relief is realized and remains continuous for several months, the dosage can be titrated down until symptoms return and discontinued entirely if no relapse is experienced at the lower dosage.

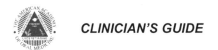
With many medications, the patient may experience several days of drowsiness initially before the drowsiness gradually wears off. During the period of time the patient is experiencing drowsiness, the patient should refrain from driving or other endeavors requiring attention.

TABLE 5 - 1: SUMMARY OF DRUGS OF CHOICE TO TREAT CHRONIC FACIAL PAIN

Medication	Available Dosages	Frequency	Notes
Drugs used topically to treat chronic pain			
EMLA cream	30 g tube	tid – qid	Apply to affected area tid. Eutectic mixture of lidocaine 2.5% and prilocaine 2.5%
Capsaicin	0.025 or 0.075% 30 g tube	tid – qid	
Clonazepam	0.5 mg tablets		Dissolve tablet in mouth or chew and rinse with mixture of tablet and saliva for 1 min
Systemic agents – tricyclic antidepressants			
Amitriptyline (Elavil)	10, 25 mg	10 – 75 mg qd	Start with 1 tablets qhs. If no response increase dose or add a daytime dose. See text above
Nortrityline (Pamelor)	10, 25 mg	10 – 75 mg qd	
Doxepin (Sinequan)	10, 25, 50, 100 mg	75 – 150 mg qd	
Systemic agents – miscellaneous categories			
Desyrel (Trazodone)	50, 100 mg	150 mg qd	
Tramadol (Ultram)	50 mg	100 mg qid maximum	Although not as addictive as many other controlled substances, the potential for abuse exists. This should not be used in patients with a history of seizures or those taking antidepressant drugs and is considered proseizure.
Sertraline (Zoloft)	25, 50, 100 mg	100 - 150 mg qd	
Paroxetine (Paxil)	10, 20 , 30, 40 mg	30 – 70 mg qd	
Mexiletine (Mexitil)	200 mg	tid	
OxyContin	10, 20, 40, 80, 160 mg		Controlled-release form of oxycodone. High abuse potential but demonstrated efficacy in long-term pain treatment.
Systemic agents – benzodiazepines			
Clonazepam	0.5, 1.0 mg	0.5 – 2 mg	Start with 1 tablets qhs. Depending on response and sedation, increase dose.
Systmeic agents – anticonvulsants			
Carbamazepine (Tegretol)	100 , 200 mg	200 – 1,200 mg qd (divided dose)	Dose titrated to effect. Start with one pill bid and depending on response and side effects; slowly increase up to 1,200 mg daily.
Phenytoin (Dilantin)	100 mg	tid	
Gabapentin (Neurontin)	300 mg	900 – 3,600 mg (divided)	

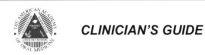

6 – LOCAL ANESTHETICS

Local anesthesia may represent the most important advance in clinical dentistry. Since virtually all dental procedures are associated with some degree of pain (or is it "discomfort"?), anesthetics make it possible to accomplish treatment that would otherwise be impossible on a conscious human being. All told, local anesthetics are probably the drugs most frequently administered by most dental practitioners. The quick onset, predictable efficacy, and tremendous margin of safety have made anesthesia a part of almost every dental visit that is not a routine prophylaxis. However, some considerations and controversies associated with these drugs bear further description.

TYPES OF ANESTHETICS

Two broad categories of anesthetics exist: esters and amides. The ester anesthetics were the original, and, for a period of time, only form of the drugs available. The most common form of this was novocaine, a name that is now virtually synonymous with local anesthesia itself. The production of ester anesthetics was largely discontinued when it was found that many individuals had allergies to para-aminobenzoic acid (PABA), a breakdown product of these drugs. Most anesthetics are now of the amide class and few individuals demonstrate true allergies to these chemicals.

INGREDIENTS IN ANESTHETICS

Anesthetics contain one or more of the following ingredients:

- Anesthetic agent. This is the actual chemical (e.g., lidocaine, mepivicaine, articaine) that produces anesthesia. All anesthetics exert their effect by impeding the flow of sodium ions across nerve membranes, thereby reducing nerve conduction.
- Vasoconstrictor. Some anesthetics include a vasoconstrictor, which serves to prolong the action of the anesthetic and decrease systemic absorption (and thereby toxicity). These chemicals also give the added bonus of aiding in local hemostasis because all anesthetics (with the exception of cocaine!) are intrinsically vasodilators. The vasoconstrictors most often used are usually epinephrine (1:50,000, 1:100,000 or 1:200,000) or levonordefrin (1:20,000). The various concentrations of vasoconstrictor differ only in the hemostatic potential that they provide and do not impact the onset, efficacy, or duration of anesthesia.
- Preservative. Sodium metabisulfite is commonly used to stabilize the degradation of the vasoconstrictor in solution.
- Buffers. Various buffering agents are used to achieve the desired pH.
- Dosing. Most anesthetics are used to achieve the desired effect in limited quantities that are significantly below the maximum dosage. However, toxic effects can manifest when excessive amounts are used. These are detailed in Table 6-1.

Vasoconstrictors. The greatest controversy surrounding anesthetics relates to the use of vasoconstrictors. Questions have arisen as to the safety of vasoconstrictor agents in individuals with certain health concerns, most notably cardiac disease and hypertension. As a general rule, it is safe to use vasoconstrictors in up to 3.6 cc of anesthetic (two carpules) with 1:100,000 epinephrine or equivalent. However, clinicians should bear in mind that most studies demonstrate increased pain control from anesthetics with vasoconstrictors. Pain is a more likely instigator of a cardiac event (via production of endogenous catecholamines) than exogenously administered epinephrine. Therefore, the additional pain control is of great value and may counter intuitively enhance safety. If there is a question as to safety, a small amount of anesthetic (one-half cartridge) can be given and vital signs monitored. If there is no change within 5 minutes, additional amounts may be slowly titrated to effect. Finally, there are rare instances in which vasoconstrictors are absolutely contraindicated, which are described in this chapter.

Allergy. Patients may state that they have had allergic reactions to local anesthetics. These are often cited as becoming "jittery," sweatiness, or nervousness. These are often truly the effects of the vasoconstrictor, and it may be worthwhile to try an anesthetic without a vasoconstrictor. If the patient describes a true allergy (e.g., swelling, rash, anaphylaxis), then it may be worthwhile to investigate if the allergy is to sulfite or the sodium metabisulfite preservative agent. Since the preservative is used only to stabilize the vasoconstrictor, selecting an agent without a vasoconstrictor may again prove helpful,

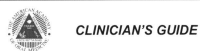
although anesthesia may be less profound. If a patient proves legitimately allergic to an amide anesthetic, another amide can be used because there seems to be little cross-allergenicity between amide molecules. In some circumstances, it is possible to use injectable diphenhydramine to achieve anesthesia as has been described in the literature.

Recently, it has become possible to reverse the effects of oral anesthesia, thereby shortening the duration of anesthesia. A formulation of phentolamine mesylate (Oraverse, Novalar pharmaceuticals, San Diego, CA) provides anti-alpha adrenergic activity and reverses the activity of vasoconstrictors. The drug may reduce duration of anesthesia by as much as 50%. Side effects, though rare, included tachycardia, bradycardia, and arrhythmia.

TABLE 6 - 1: SUMMARY OF DRUGS OF CHOICE FOR LOCAL ANESTHESIA

Name & Vasoconstrictor Options	Maximum Safe Dosage	Duration (min) (Mandibular Block)		Duration (min) (Maxilla)	
		Pulpal	Soft Tissue	Pulpal	Soft Tissue
Amide anesthetics with vasoconstrictors					
Lidocaine 2% (Xylocaine) 1:100,000 & 1:50,000 epinephrine	7 mg/kg (500 mg maximum)	85	190	60	170
Mepivivcaine 2% (Carbocaine) 1:20,000 levonordefrin	6.6 mg/kg (400 mg maximum)	75	185	50	130
Bupivicaine 0.5% (Marcaine) 1:200,000 epinephrine	2.0 mg/kg (200 mg maximum)	240	440	40	340
Prilocaine 4% (Citanest)* 1:200,000 epinephrine	8 mg/kg (500 mg maximum)	60	220	40	140
Articaine 4% (Septocaine) 1:100,000 & 1:200,000 epinephrine	7 mg/kg (500 mg maximum)	90	230	60	190
Amide anesthetics without vasoconstrictor					
Prilocaine 4% (Citanest)	8 mg/kg (500 mg maximum)	55	190	20	105
Mepivicanie 3% (Carbocaine)	6.6 mg/kg (400 mg maximum)	40	165	25	90

* Prilocaine carries the risk of methemoglobinemia if maximum dose is exceeded.

CONTRAINDICATIONS FOR USING ANESTHETIC WITH VASOCONSTRICTORS IN DENTAL PATIENTS

- Patients with stage II hypertension
- Patients with hyperthyroidism who are inadequately treated or demonstrate signs of the condition

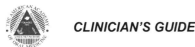
7 – ANTIBIOTIC PROPHYLAXIS

The movement of bacteria from the oral cavity to the systemic circulation is a common event, but there is a longstanding concern about the potential for a bacteremia to cause distant site infections such as infective endocarditis (IE), These concerns led to the American Heart Association (AHA) recommendations for prophylactic antibiotics, and this has been a standard of care for over 50 years in the US. These recommendations are based on the belief that invasive dental procedures cause enough of a bacteremia to put some cardiac patient populations at risk for IE. The concern about distant site infections prompted the development of similar recommendations for patients with prosthetic joints, and over 20 other medical conditions and devices have been informally recommended for prophylaxis in spite of the lack of data to show efficacy.

CARDIAC PATIENTS

The most recent AHA recommendations for the dental management of patients with cardiac abnormalities define patients at risk (Table 7-1), the dental procedures most likely to put patients at risk (Table 7-2), and the appropriate antibiotic regimen (Table 7-3). These 2007 recommendations contain significant modifications from the preceeding 1997 recommendations.

PATIENTS WITH PROSTHETIC JOINTS

In 1997, a committee representing the American Dental Association (ADA) and the American Academy of Orthopaedic Surgeons (AAOS) defined specific orthopedic joint populations at risk, and the dental procedures that put these patients at risk. This document states that "it is advisable to consider" antibiotic coverage for specific patient populations (Table 7-4). The committee adopted the 1997 AHA recommendations relative to high risk dental procedures, and the suggested antibiotic regimens, although the AHA never intended that their recommendations be used for non-cardiac patients. These ADA/AAOS recommendations were updated in 2003, and another update is anticipated in 2008. A recent opinion statement from a committee of the American Association of Orthopaedic Surgeons has essentially reversed the 1997/2003 guidelines, stating that virtually all joint patients be considered for antibiotic prophylaxis. This has sparked considerable concern in the dental arena.

TABLE 7 - 1: CARDIAC CONDITIONS ASSOCIATED WITH THE HIGHEST RISK OF ADVERSE OUTCOME FROM ENDOCARDITIS FOR WHICH PROPHYLAXIS WITH DENTAL PROCEDURES IS REASONABLE

- Prosthetic cardiac valve or prosthetic material used for cardiac valve repair
- Previous infective endocarditis
- Congenital heart disease (CHD)*
- Unrepaired cyanotic congenital heart disease, including those with palliative shunts and conduits
- Completely repaired CHD with prosthetic material or device either by surgery or catheter intervention during the first 6 months after the procedure**
- Repaired CHD with residual defects at the site or adjacent to the site of a prosthetic patch or prosthetic device (which inhibit endothelialization)
- Cardiac transplantation recipients who develop cardiac valvulopathy

* Except for the conditions listed above, antibiotic prophylaxis is no longer recommended for any other form of CHD
** Prophylaxis is reasonable because endothelialization of prosthetic material occurs within 6 months after the procedure

---

TABLE 7 - 2: DENTAL PROCEDURES FOR WHICH ENDOCARDITIS PROPHYLAXIS IS REASONABLE FOR PATIENTS IN TABLE 7 - 1

All dental procedures that involve manipulation of gingival tissue or the periapical region of teeth or perforation of the oral mucosa*

* The following procedures and events do not need prophylaxis: routine anesthetic injections through noninfected tissue, taking dental radiographs, placement of removable prosthodontic or orthodontic appliances, adjustment of orthodontic appliances, placement of orthodontic brackets, shedding of deciduous teeth and bleeding from trauma to the lips or oral mucosa.

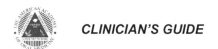
TABLE 7 - 3: REGIMENS FOR A DENTAL PROCEDURE

Situation	Agent	Regimen - Single Dose 30–60 minutes before procedure	
		Adults	**Children**
Oral	Amoxicillin	2 gm	50 mg/kg
Unable to take oral medication	Ampicillin **OR**	2 g IM or IV	50 mg/kg IM or IV
	Cefazolin **OR** ceftriaxone	1 g IM or IV	50 mg/kg IM or IV
Oral, allergic to penicillins or ampicillin	Cephalexin*† **OR**	2 g	50 m/kg
	Clindamycin **OR**	600 mg	20 mg/kg
	Azithromycin **OR** clarithromycin	500 mg	15 mg/kg
Allergic to penicillins or ampicillin and unable to take oral medication	Cefazolin **OR** ceftriaxone†	1 g IM or IV	50 mg/kg IM or IV
	OR Clindamycin phosphate	600 mg IM or IV	20 mg/kg IM or IV

IM = intramuscular; IV = intravenous.

* Or other first or second generation oral cephalosporin in equivalent adult or pediatric dosage.

† Cephalosporins should not be used in an individual with a history of anaphylaxis, angioedema, or urticaria with penicillins or ampicillin

TABLE 7 - 4: PATIENTS AT POTENTIAL RISK OF HEMATOGENOUS TOTAL JOINT INFECTION

Immunocompromised / Immunosuppressed Patients
- Inflammatory arthropathies: rheumatoid arthritis, systemic lupus erythematosus
- Disease-, drug-, or radiation-induced immunosuppression

Other Patients
- Insulin-dependent (Type 1) diabetes
- First 2 years following joint placement
- Previous prosthetic joint infections
- Malnourishment
- Hemophilia

NOTE: For dental procedures that are suggested for prophylaxis, see Table 7-2, because the dental procedures are the same as those suggested for endocarditis prophylaxis.

TABLE 7 - 5: SUGGESTED ANTIBIOTIC PROPHYLAXIS REGIMENS FOR ORTHOPAEDIC PATIENTS

Patients Not Allergic to Penicillin: Cephalexin, Cephradine, or Amoxicillin
- 2 grams orally 1 hour prior to dental procedure

Patients Not Allergic to Penicillin and Unable to Take Oral Medications: Cefazolin or Ampicillin
- 2 g intramuscularly or intravenously (IV) 1 hour prior to the procedure

Patients Allergic to Penicillin: Clindamycin
- 600 milligrams orally 1 hour prior to the dental procedure

Patients Allergic to Penicillin and Unable to Take Oral Medications: Clindamycin
- 600 mg IV 1 hour prior to the procedure

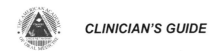

8 – TREATMENT OF ANXIETY

For many patients, the mere idea of a dental visit is one of the most anxietycausing thoughts they can have. For simple or, at times, complex psychological reasons, some patients cannot relax and let the dental professionals begin and complete their work. Other patients, because of recent or long-standing physiologic compromise, such as previous heart attack or hypertension, may appear calm, but may experience serious consequences if provoked into anxiety. For both patient categories, there are a number of available agents, from over-the-counter medications (OTCs) to controlled substances from which the clinician may choose that can sedate or relax the patient. In all cases, one should be methodical and start with the mildest medication based on the assessment of each individual patient. Perhaps the most effective sedation may be a quiet chairside manner and thorough explanation of all procedures.

The least sedating drugs, which prove adequate under many circumstances, are antihistamines. Diphenhydramine (Benadryl) is an OTC medication supplied in several dosage forms. Hydroxyzine (Atarax) is an antihistamine/antiemetic with an established history as a safe, mild sedating agent. Physiologic effects of antihistamines include sedation and a bonus of xerostomia. Dosages and notes are given in the following table.

The drugs of choice today are the controlled substances collectively known as the benzodiazepines (BDZs). As a group, they demonstrate the following effects: sedation, skeletal muscle relaxation, anxiolysis, and anticonvulsive activity. They also carry the risk of mild habituation. The 16 to 18 medications in this large group in the United States vary widely in the selective expression of the above properties as well as in half-life. Of the 18 agents available, 3 or perhaps 4 are best suited as preappointment sedating medications for dental patients. These are chosen because they offer adequate sedation with few side effects and relatively short and finite half lives. Serax (oxazepam), Ativan (lorazepam), and Xanax (alprazolam) are included. Valium (diazepam), which has an extremely long half-life, is included simply because of its long track record, public familiarity, and availability of multiple preparations. All of these benzodiazepines may be taken the day of the appointment, as well as combined with an additional dose at bed-time the night prior to the day of the appointment to help ensure a worry-free night's sleep. All BDZs listed here are available in multiple strengths. A good rule of thumb is to start patients on the middle dosage available. It may also be useful to give patients an additional dose or two of the medication so that they can "test" their response prior to the preappointment scenario. This minimizes the risk of an inadequate response on the day of dental visit. All BDZs are contraindicated in pregnant patients.

The most powerful sedative-hypnotic short of intravenous conscious sedation methods may be the barbiturate class. Secobarbital is a short- to intermediateonset and duration drug that was quite popular for preoperative dental sedation some years ago. The barbiturates as a class, however, have numerous drawbacks including habituation, numerous drug interactions, and respiratory depression. However, when used infrequently, in limited doses, and in a controlled fashion, barbiturates represent a viable alternative to benzodiazepines for sedation.

Table 8 – 1 on the next page lists the drugs of choice to control anxiety prior to dental visits.

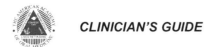
TABLE 8 - 1: DRUGS OF CHOICE TO TREAT ANXIETY			
Sedative Agent	*Available Preparations (mg)*	*Half-Life (hr)*	*Notes*
Antihistamines			
Diphenhydramine (Benadryl)	25 – 30	6	OTC, very inexpensive, xerostomic
Hydroxyzine (Atarax)	25 – 100	3	Requires prescription, antiemetic and xerostomic activity
Benzodiazepines (Schedule IV)			
Oxazepam (Serax)	10, 15, 30	4 – 14	Finite, should be given 2 h prior to appointment owing to slower onset
Lorazepam (Ativan)	0.5, 1, 2	10 -20	Liquid available
Alprazolam (Xanax)	0.25, 0.5, 1, 2	6 – 20	Finite, liquid available, most habit forming benzodiazepine
Diazepam (Valium)	2, 5, 10	20 – 90	Not finite, effect too long, longer in females and elderly
Barbiturates (Schedule II)			
Secobarbital (Seconal)	25, 50, 100	28	Hangover effects, more habituation than benzodiazepines, last resort before conscious sedation techniques

OTC = over-the- counter

Notes:

- Sedatives are typically dosed 1 hour prior to start of appointment.
- Patients are required to have someone provide transportation for them to and from the appointment.
- It is often helpful to have the patient take an additional dose 1 hour prior to bedtime the night before the day of treatment.

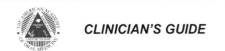
9 – TREATMENT OF VESICULAR / EROSIVE DISEASES

Oral vesiculoerosive diseases (OVED), comprising of oral lichen planus (OLP), mucous membrane pemphigoid (MMP), pemphigus vulgaris (PV), epidermolysis bullosa acquisita (EBA) and erythema multiforme (EM), are considered to have an autoimmune etiology. Differential diagnosis of such lesions include viral infections, fungal infections, periodontal disease, systemic disorders (e.g.: systemic lupus erythematosus), contact reactions to oral materials (e.g.: amalgam, methyl methacrylate) and reactions to medications (e.g.: lichenoid reactions).

The correct diagnosis must first be established through a thorough history, clinical examination, tissue biopsy followed by histopathological analysis, and laboratory tests, when indicated. Once a correct diagnosis is established, the therapeutic approach varies according to the disease and its severity.

This chapter outlines treatment guidelines for OVED based upon the disease diagnosis, severity and extent. By no means is this an all encompassing list of all conditions and medications. The dosages herein are not to simply be followed as "recipes," as the patient's medical history, response to therapeutics and adverse side effects should all be considered along with these treatment guidelines. Medications function as 'tools' for patients to control their signs and symptoms, since these chronic diseases cannot be cured. This chapter does not address oral lesions from systemic disorders and reactive lesions from drugs and materials.

Many cases of OVED can be managed solely with topical or systemic steroids. Depending on severity, response and side effects, other immunosuppressive medications or agents, either alone, or in combination with steroids, can be tried. If the practitioner does not feel comfortable working with any of these drugs, they may refer their patient to a specialist who has more experience using them. Patients should be followed closely and regularly once therapy starts, whether it is systemic or topical therapy, to monitor disease response and side effects associated with treatment.

Steps in the diagnosis and management of OVED:

1. Obtain a thorough history from the patient.
2. Rule out a drug, herb, or dental material as the cause of their oral lesions. Ask the patient if there were any new drug, herb or dental material that was introduced within the last 6 months. Look for correlation between such changes and the onset or exacerbation of the oral condition. If you suspect a medication, call the patient's primary care physician to discuss your concerns and request that they may consider a substitute drug.
3. Determine whether the clinical course is acute or chronic. EM generally has an acute onset whereas OLP, MMP and PV and EBA are chronic.
4. Perform a thorough clinical examination. Take note of the extent (localized versus generalized), size and location, and presence or absence of the Nikolsky sign.
5. If an OVED is suspected, perform a biopsy. The biopsy should consist of lesional tissue placed in formalin for H&E staining, and perilesional tissue placed in Michel's solution for direct immunofluorescence (DIF).
6. Obtain laboratory tests, if indicated. Blood tests looking for serum antibodies (indirect immunofluorescence [IIF]) are diagnostic for PV.
7. When you receive all results and obtain a diagnosis, review the results and likely prognosis with the patient. Discuss treatment of signs and symptoms of disease. The patient needs to understand that therapies may be required over an extended period of time for disease control, and that for most OVED, there is no cure. The patient's understanding of their disease and its medical management is crucial for success.
8. Address oral hygiene and oral care. The patient should proceed with comprehensive dental care, comprising of a thorough examination and cleaning. If the patient is uncomfortable with dental treatment due to their OVED, they may defer their treatment until after their disease is controlled.

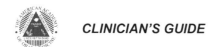

TABLE 9 – 1: DRUGS OF CHOICE IN TREATMENT OF OVED

Drugs	*Notes*	*Dosages*
Topical Corticosteroids		
Ointments: Clobetasol 0.05% Fluocinonide 0.05%	Use custom trays if disease is confined to the palate or gingival mucosa. Use moistened cotton rolls for gingival, labial and buccal mucosae.	Apply to affected areas for up to 5 – 10 minutes bid - tid.
Rinse: Dexamethasone 0.5 mg / ml elixir	Indicated for palatal or widespread lesions.	Rinse 1 teaspoonful (5 ml) for 1 - 2 minutes then expectorate bid - tid.
Other topical agents		
Tacrolimus 0.1% ointment (Protopic)	Use custom trays or moistened cotton rolls if indicated. FDA Black Box warning of a theoretical increased risk of malignancy.	Apply to affected areas for up to 5 – 10 minutes tid.
Systemic Corticosteroids		
Prednisone	AM administration so as to not affect circadian rhythms. Long-term use may exacerbate or initiate complications in patients with: diabetes, hypertension, osteoporosis, immune deficiencies, psychiatric and mood disorders. Medication must be withdrawn gradually, tapering doses over several weeks.	*Induction Therapy:* 1.0 – 2.5 mg / kg / day (50 – 80 mg qd) until 50 – 75% remission of signs and symptoms (average time 2-6 weeks) *Maintenance Therapy (Disease 80% Control):* Start to phase down to lower doses. Consider combining with systemic immunosuppresants (e.g.: azathioprine, MMF) to decrease steroid dose.
Other systemic agents		
Tetracycline	Associated with photosensitivity. Caution in patients on warfarin.	500 mg bid.
Dapsone	Side effects: hemolysis, methemoglobinemia, serum sickness Contraindicated in patients with glucose-6-phosphate dehydrogenase deficiency (G6PD) and other hemolytic anemias.	Get G6PD screen and CBC prior to therapy. Start at 25 mg qd. Taper up by 25 mg q 3 days. Target dose: 100 – 200 mg qd. Regular monitoring of CBC.
Azathioprine (Imuran)	Side effects: Nausea / vomiting; marrow aplasia A thiopurine methyltransferase (TPMT) assay performed prior to initiating.	Initial dose 1.0 mg / kg / d (50 – 100 mg). Gradually increase in 0.5 mg / kg/ d increments over several weeks. Maximum dose 2 mg / kg / d. Regular monitoring of CBC.
Mycophenolate mofetil (Cell Cept)	An alternative agent for those who are unable to tolerate azathioprine.	35 – 45 mg / kg / d

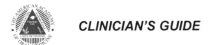
TABLE 9 – 2: KEY FEATURES AND TREATMENT STRATEGIES FOR OVED		
Disease	**Diagnostic Features**	**Treatment Strategy**
Oral Lichen Planus (OLP)	Chronic, multiple ulcerations Erythema with white plaques or striae Biopsy necessary to rule out MMP, PV, SLE and dysplasia or malignancy Histopathology – Hyperkeratosis, band-like infiltrate of lymphocytes	*Mild to moderate:* Topical corticosteroids as first line treatment Topical tacrolimus only as second-line therapy. *Severe, wide-spread:* Systemic corticosteroids; Azathioprine
Mucous Membrane Pemphigoid (MMP)	Desquamative gingivitis along with other mucosal surfaces Positive Nicolsky sign May have ocular involvement Histopathology – Subepithelial clefting DIF – Autoantibodies at basement membrane Salt-split test – Autoantibodies on the roof of bulla IIF – Negative	*Mild:* Topical corticosteroids as first line treatment, intralesional steroids *Moderate, severe or refractory:* Tetracycline; Dapsone; Systemic corticosteroids; Azathioprine
Pemphigus Vulgaris (PV)	Mucocutaneous and skin involvement Positive Nicolsky sign Histopathology – Intraepithelial clefting DIF – Autoantibodies in the basal epithelium IIF – Positive	Systemic corticosteroids as first line treatment. Dapsone, Azathioprine, MMF Intralesional steroids IV gammaglobulin
Epidermolysis bullosa acquisita (EBA)	Oral and skin lesions. Histopathology – Subepithelial clefting DIF – Autoantibodies at basement membrane Salt-split test – Autoantibodies on the floor of bulla	Systemic corticosteroids as first line treatment. Dapsone, Azathioprine, MMF
Erythema Multiforme (EM)	Acute, multiple lesions and deep ulcers May have precipitating factor (e.g.: infection, drugs) Affects skin and mucosa – lip crusting, 'target lesions' on skin Spares the gingiva Histopathology – Subepithelial edema and perivascular inflammation	Symptomatic relief only for mild cases Systemic corticosteroids Prophylaxis against herpes simplex virus if presumed cause (see Chapter 2) Discontinuance of suspected precipitating drugs

Notes:

- Avoid food known to irritate the mouth.

- Avoid antimicrobial mouth rinses such as chlorhexidine, and Listerine® due to alcohol content.

- Monitor patient for oral candidal infection while on topical or systemic corticosteroids. Consider prescribing antifungal medications as an adjunct for all on topical or systemic corticosteroids (see Chapter 3).

10 – PHARMACOLOGIC MANAGEMENT OF DENTAL CARIES

Current research documents that dental decay is an infectious disease associated with pathogenic biofilm dominated by specific organisms, specifically, lactobacilli, mutans streptococci group and other low pH non-mutans streptococci bacteria. Risk factors associated with higher rates of caries formation include:

- Gingival recession (leading to demineralization of softer root surfaces)

- Salivary hypofunction (often associated with medications that reduce salivary flow)

- Diet high in fermentable sugars (sucrose)

- Poor oral hygiene (In the elderly, this is often associated with impaired manual dexterity.)

TREATMENT

For non-cavitated surfaces, depending on the location, extent of decay, and activity of the lesion chemical remineralization procedures may be preferred. When surface cavitation and bacterial invasion is present in the dentin, the infected dentin must be surgically removed (ie, cavity preparation) and the missing tooth structure replaced with restorative materials. For decay on the roots a fluoride containing restorative material such as glass ionomer may and perhaps should be considered. Once the active decay is removed and the teeth restored, treatment should be directed at preventing further decay.

Caries Prevention for Low- and Medium-Risk Patients

1. Oral hygiene instruction, to keep down the number of organisms.

2. Dietary counseling to decrease the frequency of consumption of fermentable carbohydrates.

3. Apply fluoride to "harden the teeth," more specifically, it inhibits demineralization, facilitates remineralization, and inhibits bacterial growth.

    a. Fluoride is available in a variety of formulations and concentrations. The choice of which fluoride to use depends on the severity of decay and resources available to the patient.

    b. The fluoride concentrations (in parts per million [ppm]) available include:

      225 ppm over-the-counter (OTC) rinses
      1,000 to 1,500 ppm OTC toothpastes
      5,000 ppm Rx gels, toothpastes, and a rinse
      9,000 to 12,000 ppm gels and foams used in dental offices
      22,600 ppm fluoride varnish

4. Use an OTC fluoride-containing toothpaste after each meal.

5. Use an OTC fluoride-containing rinse between meals or if the patient is not able to brush.

Caries Prevention for High-Risk Patients

Caries prevention in high-risk patients (those with a lot of decay) requires the above prevention strategies as well as the use of high-concentration fluorides and specific therapy directed at treating the infection that is the cause of the decay.

Treatment to strengthen the teeth:

Prescribe high-concentration fluoride toothpaste.

If necessary, in lieu of the above or because of inadequate caries reduction with the above prescription toothpaste, construct a custom fluoride tray to use to apply a high-concentration fluoride gel.

If possible, fluoride varnish should be applied to the patient's teeth once every 3-4 months. In many patients, because of an inability to comply with other treatment options, fluoride varnish may be the best and only option.

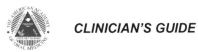
Treatment to control the infection:

No matter what approach you have used relative to fluoride, high-risk patients should also be treated to control the infection of dental decay. One or all of the approaches in Table 10-1 could be used. Recently, research has suggested that a low pH in the mouth selects for a pathogenic (acidic) biofilm and therefore by raising the pH it not only selects for a healthy biofilm but also promotes remineralization (see www.carifree.com).

Treatment for abnormal saliva:

Saliva is the most important protective factor and when there is any abnormality (low resting pH, inadequate buffering capacity, salivary gland hypofunction/xerotomia) it must be countered chemically with products that neutralize acid and provide a source of calcium and phosphate.

TABLE 10 – 1: AGENTS USED IN TREATMENT OF CARIES

Agent	Quantity	Instructions
Management of Infectious Aspect of Caries Process		
Chlorhexidine0.12% rinse	16 oz bottle (prescription only)	Rinse with 1 tbsp (15 mL) bid for 1 week. Repeat once a month until bacterial levels drop.
CariFree Treatment Rinse	Comes in a two bottle (A & B)rinse www.carifree.com	Rinse with 1 tbsp (15 mL) of rinse A and B bid for 2 weeks followed by user of CariFree Maintenance Rinse for 2 weeks. Repeat once a month until bacterial levels drop.
Xylitol* gum or candy	100 pieces (available OTC) www.xclear.com www.xylitol.org	Chew 1 gum or suck on 1 candy for 5 minutes 5-10 times a day. Discontinue gum and switch to candy if TMJ or muscular problems occur.
Fluoride Agents		
PreviDent 5000 Plus Or any 5000 ppm fluoride containing toothpaste. There are many brands.	2 oz tube	Brush thoroughly for 2 min daily, preferably at bedtime. Spit only; do not rinse. Nothing to eat or drink for 30 min.
Neutral NaF gel 1.1% (5,000 ppm)	2 oz tube	1 drop per tooth in custom-made trays. Wear for 3–5 min each day. Nothing to eat or drink for 30 min.
Fluoride varnish All contain 22,600 ppm NaFl		Apply varnish to patient's teeth every 3-6 months at routine prophylaxis visit.
pH Agents		
CariFree Boost Salese/Dentiva	www.carifree.com www.nuvorainc.com/	Spray into mouth throughout the day as needed
Calcium/phosphate Agents		
CPP – ACP (MI Paste/Recaldent ACP (ADA Foundation) CSP (Novamin)	The listed produces are in a variety of different dental products	
TCP (Tri Calcium Phosphate)		

* Xylitol must be the predominate sugar in any effective product. Not all products that contain xylitol have it in a high enough concentration to be effective. For more information, see http://www.xylitol.org.

OTC = over-the-counter; TMJ = temporomandibular joint.

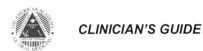
11 – DRUG INTERACTIONS

Drugs interfere with other drugs because of both pharmacokinetics and pharmacodynamics. Pharmacokinetics refers to the movement through the body's various systems. Pharmacokinetic principles include absorption, distribution, and elimination (what the body does to the drug). Pharmacodynamics refers to the function of drugs with regard to receptors and receptor systems (what the drug does to the body).

The therapeutic window is the dosage between the minimal dose at which the drug is effective and the dose at which drug toxicity begins. Some drugs such as antibiotics have a large therapeutic window. These drugs are relatively safe, and it would be difficult for a patient to overdose with them. However, some drugs have a relatively narrow therapeutic window. It is important for the clinician to be careful with drugs which have narrow therapeutic windows.

Absorption drug interactions include situations in which one drug may alter the absorption kinetics of another drug. For instance, many drugs require a specific level of acidity for absorption. Therefore, drugs which alter the stomach's acidity will alter the level of absorption of many other drugs. Furthermore, some drugs may precipitate another drug out of solution, thereby limiting the ability of that drug to be absorbed by the stomach.

With regard to distribution, many drugs are attached to protein (albumin) as they travel through the bloodstream. While the drug is attached to the albumin molecule, it is not available within the serum solution as it reaches equilibrium between its attachment to the protein and its serum concentration. Another drug which has an affinity for albumin may knock the first drug off the protein and therefore increase the serum concentration of the first drug. This interaction may result in increased serum concentrations of one or both drugs, which may result in toxicity.

The main elimination pathways are twofold: renal and hepatic. Drug interactions can affect either of these processes. Some antibiotics such as penicillin are eliminated by the kidney and other drugs which influence kidney filtration or reabsorption can therefore influence the elimination of penicillin. For example, probenecid, a drug used in the treatment of gout, decreases the speed at which penicillin is eliminated, which thereby increases its duration of action.

The liver is important with regard to biotransformation, which is an important first step in the detoxification process. There are a number of hepatic biotransformation pathways, generally known as the hepatic cytochrome P450 or CYP system. These include both substrate and inhibition biochemical pathways CYP 1A2, 2C9, 2C19, 2D6, 2E1, and 3A4.

Pharmacodynamic drug interactions involve either competition for a receptor site or blockage of a receptor. As an example of this action, an agonist for the mu receptor is morphine, which may be blocked by the mu receptor antagonist naloxone. Therefore, the drug naloxone is used essentially as an antidote for morphine overdose. Also, many drugs are delivered in a prodrug or inactivated form. These drugs require activation through a biochemical action in order to be activated and therefore provide a working form of the drug. Such drugs as prednisone require bacterial enzymatic activity to produce the drug prednisolone, which is the active form of the drug.

CLASSIFICATION OF DRUG INTERACTIONS BY MECHANISM CATEGORY

Additive Interactions

Drugs with the same toxicity profile interact negatively when added together. For example, drugs such as aspirin and the antibiotic gentamicin both are noted for causing ototoxicity (hearing toxicity). Therefore, these drugs should not be used together because although using the therapeutic range for each drug individually may not reach toxic levels, the combination may reach a toxic level with regard to hearing loss. Also, drugs of the same drug category such as ibuprofen and naproxen should not be used together because they both have a similar toxicity profile, and if each drug is used within its therapeutic range,

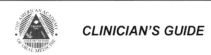
there is no problem. However, when both drugs are used at therapeutic dose levels, the toxicity level may be breached.

No Additive Toxicity

Many drug combinations are used with drugs that have similar drug actions but different toxicity profiles. These drugs may be combined so that when both drugs are used within their therapeutic ranges, there is maximal therapeutic effect and no significant increase with regard to toxicity. Examples of such combinations include acetaminophen with a narcotic or a nonsteroidal anti-inflammatory drug (NSAID) with a narcotic drug. This principal is critical to achieving increased drug action (in the example, the action would be analgesia) without increased toxicity.

Absorption Interference

Antacids or other gastric secretion–modifying agents (H2 blockers or proton pump inhibitors) may interfere with the absorption of drugs such as aspirin or ketoconazole which require stomach acidity for absorption. Drugs or substances rich in calcium or divalent cations (eg, some antacids) may interfere with a drug known for the chelation of calcium such as the antibiotic tetracycline. The tetracycline binds to the calcium (or sometimes to another bivalent molecule) and the chelation complex is precipitated out and therefore not absorbed.

Enzyme Induction

Some drugs such as alcohol, barbiturates, theophylline, anticonvulsants, and antibiotic drugs such as rifampin may speed up the biotransformation process. Because rifampin has the potential to increase the biotransformation and elimination process of oral contraceptives, it is the only antibiotic proven to interfere with contraception.

Enzyme Inhibition

Some drugs such as cimetidine, diazepam, digoxin, and isoniazid may interfere with the biotransformation process resulting in decreased speed of elimination and increased serum drug levels of other drugs, possibly resulting in toxicity.

Protein Bumping

Drugs which have affinity for protein (albumin) binding may knock one another off of the protein molecule resulting in higher serum concentrations of other drugs known to be protein bound. Such drugs as NSAIDs, coumadin, aspirin, oral hypoglycemics, and phenytoin are known to be protein bound. If the patient is taking one of these drugs, then adding another one has the potential to increase drug serum levels of one or both drugs.

Competitive Inhibition

Drugs have various biochemical biotransformation pathways (cytochrome isoforms 1A2, 2C9, 2C19, 2D6, 2E1, and 3A4) and in cases where more than one drug competes for a particular pathway, the elimination process may be decreased.

Macrolide Drug Interactions

The macrolides (erythromycin, theophylline, H1 blockers [terfenadine, cisapride], coumadin, carbamazepine, corticosteroids, cyclosporine, digoxin, ketoconazole, propoxyphene, and statins) have common biotransformation pathways (1A2 and 3A4). Taking any two of these drugs may result in competitive inhibition, increased serum concentrations of one or more drugs, and the potential for toxicity.

Monoamine Oxidase Inhibitor Drug Interactions

Monoamine oxidase (MAO) inhibitors are known to interact with several drugs with the possibility of a severe hypertensive crisis due to immediate neurotransmitter release. Drugs such as meperidine are absolutely contraindicated for patients taking MAO inhibitors.

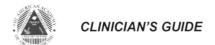
TABLE 11 – 1: NOTABLE DRUG INTERACTIONS WITH RESPECT TO DENTISTRY		
Drug	*Other Drug*	*Interaction Result*
Aspirin	Gentamycin	Hearing loss
NSAID	Other NSAID	Bleeding, gastric toxicity
NSAID	Coumadin	Bleeding
Acetaminophen	Ethyl alcohol	Liver toxicity
Narcotic	Other narcotic	Respiratory depression
Meperidine	MAO inhibitor	Hypertension
Tramadol	SSRIs	Seizure
Local anesthetic	Other local anesthetic	Arrhythmia
Local anesthetic	Cocaine	Arrhythmia
Erythromycin	Theophylline	Arrhythmia
Erythromycin	Coumadin	Bleeding
Erythromycin	Carbamazepine	Liver toxicity
Ketoconazole	Quinidine	Arrhythmia
Ketoconazole	Theophylline	Arrhythmia
Metronidiazole	Alcohol	Headache/nausea/vomiting

MAO = monoamine oxidase; NSAID = nonsteroidal anti-inflammatory drug; SSRI = selective serotonin reuptake inhibitor.

Notes:

1. Vasoconstrictors within local anesthetic formulations have been purported to interact with tricyclic antidepressants and nonselective β-blockers. However, scientific evidence does not presently support these contentions.

2. Broad-spectrum antibiotics have been purported to interfere with the activation of birth control pills, thereby decreasing the efficacy of birth control; however, the scientific evidence does not presently support this contention.

3. There are many more drug-drug interactions that are possible. It is incumbent upon clinicians to consider possible interactions with any prescribed drug and even alternative and over-the-counter products. For further information, it may be necessary to consult the Physicians Desk Reference (PDR) or a pharmacology text.

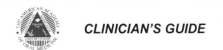
12 – COMPLEMENTARY AND ALTERNATIVE MEDICINES

Natural, holistic, alternative, and *traditional* are all terms which refer to medical practices not taught in Western medical schools. These practices are now grouped under Complementary and Alternative Medicine (CAM). CAM is also referred to as integrative medicine. There are CAM compounds available for virtually all human ailments.

There is a perception, especially in Western medicine, that there is relatively little scientific, evidence-based documentation of the efficacy of these compounds, but that is not true. There is a wealth of such information available from reputable sources (see Chapter 18), documenting the efficacy and safety of CAM products. There are also a growing number of reputable harvesters/manufacturers of consistently high-quality products and a growing integration of CAM into Western medical practice. This is driven in part by patients who want more natural wellness-based (as opposed to disease-based) therapies from their physicians and dentists.

The purpose of this chapter is to introduce you to some of the best CAM products for oral health problems.

If you would like to develop a better understanding of the broad range of such phytomedicines (Gr. *phyto* = plant) and CAM products, an excellent book on the topic is **The Green Pharmacy** by James A. Duke. From such a reading, you will better appreciate the preventive nature of CAM products and therapies, a common focus of dental practice. The best, most comprehensive reference on CAM products is *Natural Medicines Comprehensive Database* published by The Pharmacist's Letter.

In this chapter, you will find CAM products to manage periodontal diseases and canker sores, herpetic ulcers, anxiety, caries, dry mouth, halitosis, and wound healing. In addition, preventive and supportive nutritional aids to enhance oral health are also covered (Table 12-1). These products particularly apply to the surgical patient.

TABLE 12 – 1: COMPLEMETARY AND ALTERNATIVE DRUGS AND SUPPLEMENTS		
Category / Product Name / Uses	*Manufacturer / Contact Informtation*	*OTC / Rx*
Bacterial Infection		
Insure Herbal Echinacea & Goldenseal Combination Extract (Antibacterial, antiviral, immunostimulant)	Zand Herbal Formulas, Inc., Ferndale, WA, 1-800-227-6063 www.nutraceutical.com	OTC
Gum Guard (Contains gram+ bacteria to prevent/displace gram bacteria–induced gingivitis and periodontal diseases; e.g., maintains/restores homeostasis.)	Gum Guard, Inc. Venice, FL,1-866-FIT-GUMS www.gumguard.com	OTC
The Natural Dentist Healthy Gums Therapy Daily Oral Rinse (pre- and post-treatment, maintain periodontal health) CAUTION: pH 3.2	Natural Dentist Inc, Medford, MA, 1-800-615-6895 www.thenaturaldentist.com	OTC
Probiotics 5 Capsules (Although promoted for gastrointestinal, reproductive and urinary tract health, healthy gram+/gram- balance intraorally also may be restored.)	Pure Encapsulations, Sudbury, MA, 1-800-753-2277, www.PureCaps.com	OTC

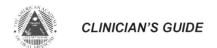
TABLE 12 – 1: COMPLEMETARY AND ALTERNATIVE DRUGS AND SUPPLEMENTS (CONTINUED)

Category / Product Name / Uses	Manufacturer / Contact Information	OTC / Rx
Viral Infection		
Lip Clear Lysine Plus + Ointment (Cold sore prevention and treatment.)	Quantum, Inc. Eugene, OR, 1-800-448-1448, www.quantumhealth.com	OTC
Herb Pharm Clove (Certified organic extract of the crimson flower buds of *Syzygium aromaticum*. 10% topically in combination with Zovirax reported to work better than either drug alone.)	Herb Pharm, Williams, OR, 1-800-348-4372, www.herb-pharm.com	OTC/ Rx
Herp-Eeze Next Generation Capsules (Stops viral replication within infected cells and prevents them from binding to healthy cells.)	Novus Research, Inc. Gilbert, AZ, 1-800-244-2438, www.phoenixlongevity.com	OTC
Sambucol Black Elderberry Original Syrup Virologist Developed (Available in lozenges. For upper respiratory health; inhibits viral entry into cells; induces sweating if feverish.)	Razei Bar Industries exclusively for Nature's Way Products Springville, UT, 1-801-489-1500, www.naturesway.com	OTC
Lemon Balm *Melissa officinalis* Capsules (When utilized during early-onset stage may mute or prevent infection; may require up to nine times the recommended dosage [Foster, S "101 Medicinal Herbs"].)	Nutraceutical Corp. exclusively for Solaray, Inc., Park City, UT, 1-800-669-8877	OTC
Fungal Infection		
Healthy Mouth Plus Natural Organic Tea Tree & Aloe Vera Gel Toothpaste (Whitens, reduces tartar build-up; fights bad breath via antimicrobial action.)	Jason Natural Cosmetics (a subsidiary of The Hain Celestial Group), Culver City, CA, 1-877-JASON-01, www.jason-natural.com	OTC
Candida Cleanse Tablets (A formula that is both preventive and therapeutic. Supports a healthy population of beneficial bacteria; energizing; easily digested.)	Rainbow Light, Santa Cruz, CA, 1-800-635-1233, ww.rainbowlight.com	OTC
Candex Capsules (A potent combination of digestive enzymes that destroys the cell wall of *Candida albicans* and digests the primary carbohydrate food sources of the organism.)	Pure Essence Labs, Las Vegas, NV, 1-888-254-8000, www.pureessencelabs.com	OTC
PROSymbiotics Colostrum Capsules Candida specific Professional Series (specific antibodies to *Candida albicans*; increases probiotic bifidobacteria; reduces bioavailability of iron to pathogens).	PROSymbiotics, Sedona, AZ, 1-888-784-4355, www.prosymbiotics.com	OTC

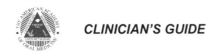

TABLE 12 – 1: COMPLEMETARY AND ALTERNATIVE DRUGS AND SUPPLEMENTS (CONTINUED)

Category / Product Name / Uses	Manufacturer / Contact Information	OTC / Rx
Antiseptic		
Tooth & Gums Tonic (Antimicrobial, tissue conditioning, connective tissue rebuilding, soothing, outstanding breath freshener.)	Dental Herb Co., Boca Raton, FL, 1-800-747-4372	OTC
Healthy Mouth Tea Tree & Cinnamon Naturally Antiseptic Mouthwash (Helps prevent bad breath, helps gums stay healthy, helps fight bacteria build-up.)	Jason Natural Cosmetics, Culver City, CA, 1-877-JASON-01, www.jason-natural.com	OTC
Pain Management (Acute)		
Gelclair Bioadherent Oral Gel Rinse (For example, mucositis, postsurgical, traumatic ulcer, ill-fitting denture, aphthous ulcer, braces-related.)	OSI Oncology Pharmacology, Melville, NY, 1-631-962-2000, www.gelclair.com	Rx
Camilia Baby Teething Homeopathic Medicine (Painful gums, restlessness, and irritability.)	Boiron-Borneman, Inc., Newton Square, PA, 1-610-325-7480 FAX	OTC
Red Cross Toothache Medication (Apply liquid topically with enclosed cotton & tweezers.) (Temporary toothache relief.) Alternate: apply whole clove to buccal mucosa adjacent tooth	The Mentholatum Co., Orchard Park, NY, 1-716-677-2500, 1-877-636-2677	OTC
Oragesic Oral Pain Reliever Irrigating solution containing *Yerba santa* (Temporary relief of minor irritation, pain, sore mouth and sore throat.)	Parnell Pharmaceuticals, Inc., San Rafael, CA, 1-800-457-4276	OTC
Anxiety/Sedation		
St. John's Wort Emotional Balance Botanical Support for Emotional Well-Being Tablets. May help support a positive emotional state, calming, supports mental health.)	Planetary Herbals, Soquel, CA, 1-800-606-6226	OTC
Oral Ulcers		
Canker Sores Begone Topical Gel (Use before or after dental appointments to provide pain relief if prone to canker sores, or whenever they occur; has herbal antiviral properties.)	Robin Barr Enterprises, Inc., Mission Viejo, CA, 1-888-877-6315, www.csbegone.com	OTC
Orahealth Cankermelts-GX Bioadherent Discs (Canker sore treatment. This product is a derivative of licorice but it is not promoted as a "natural" alternative product per se.)	Oramelts Corp. for Orahealth USA, Inc., Bellevue, WA, 1-877-672-6541	OTC

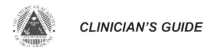
TABLE 12 – 1: COMPLEMETARY AND ALTERNATIVE DRUGS AND SUPPLEMENTS (CONTINUED)

Category / Product Name / Uses	Manufacturer / Contact Informtation	OTC / Rx
Halitosis		
Zox Mints (Breath freshener, stimulates saliva flow)	TheraBreath, Dr. Harold Katz, LLC, Los Angeles, CA, 1-800-97-FRESH	OTC
Tooth & Gums Spritz (Concentrated antiseptic mouth spray in a convenient nonaerosolized dispenser.)	Dental Herb Co., Boca Raton, FL, 1-800-747-4372	OTC
Caries Prevention		
Tooth & Gums Paste (Freshens breath, inhibits cariogenic bacterial adherence to enamel; contains anticariogenic green tea.)	Dental Herb Co., Boca Raton, FL, 1-800-747-4372	OTC
Tea Tree Oil & Neem Toothpaste with baking soda & essential oil of wintergreen, cooling mint, ginger or fennel (Freshens and cleans, reduces plaque formation.)	Desert Essence, Valencia, CA, 1-800-949-7331, www.desertessence.com	OTC
Peelu The Natural Cleansing toothpaste for a beautiful, healthy smile (Whitens and protects naturally for cleaner healthier teeth.)	Peelu Products, Ltd., The Natural Oral and Beauty Care Company, Fargo, ND, 1-800-457-3358	OTC
Spry Dental Defense System sugarfree gums—cinnamon, fresh fruit, peppermint & spearmint (Sweetened with all natural xylitol.)	Xlear Inc., Orem, UT, 1-877-599-5327, www.sprydental.com	OTC
Tom's of Maine "Natural Baking Soda Toothpaste" with fluoride peppermint (the oil from the leaf has antibacterial and antiviral properties).	Tom's Of Maine, Inc., Kennebunk, ME, 1-800-367-8867	OTC
Dry Mouth		
Thayers Dry Mouth Spray or Lozenges (Moiturize, buffer saliva, promote healthy bone, promote salivation via natural oil flavors.)	Henry Thayer Co., Westport, CT, 1-203-226-0940, www.Thayers.com	OTC
MouthKote Oral Moisturizer (Clinically proven to relieve dry mouth up to four times longer than traditional saliva substitutes; sweetened withanticariogenic xylitol.)	Parnell Pharmaceuticals, Inc, San Rafael, CA, 1-800-457-4276	OTC
Biotene Gentle Mouthwash (Antibacterial; cleans and refreshes without burning or staining; neutralizes mouth odors; promotes gingival health.)	Laclede Corp., Rancho Dominguez, CA, 1-800-922-5856	OTC

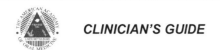

TABLE 12 – 1: COMPLEMETARY AND ALTERNATIVE DRUGS AND SUPPLEMENTS (CONTINUED)		
Category / Product Name / Uses	*Manufacturer / Contact Informtation*	*OTC / Rx*
Wound Healing		
Immunacea Certified Organic Echinacea Extract (Immunostimulant, antibacterial, antiviral.)	Tyler Encapsulations, Division of Integrative Therapeutics, Wilsonville, OR, 1-800-931-1709, www.integrativeinc.com	OTC
HerbImmune Capsules Herbal Immune Support (Facilitates healing by stimulating the immune system.)	Karuna Corp., Novato, CA, 1-800-826-7225, www.karunahealth.com	OTC
Bio-Dent (Supports bone health and protects against bone loss; may aid bone healing. Developed by Royal Lee, DDS; in use since 1955.)	Standard Process, Inc., Palmyra, WI, 1-800-848-5061	OTC
Aloe Vera Gel Made with Certified Organic Aloe Vera Leaves (The label calls for drinking the gel; alternately, apply the gel directly ontolesions to enhance healing.) Caution: pH 3.6–3.8	Lily of the Desert, Denton, TX, 1-800-229-5459, www.lilyofthedesert.com	OTC
Carlson Golden Aloe Vera Gel Concentrate (200:1) (Either swallow capsules or split open the gelcaps and apply the aloe directly to wounds to aid healing.)	Carlson Division of J.R. Carlson Laboratories, Inc., Arlington Heights, IL, 1-888-234-5656, www.carlsonlabs.com (An FDA Regulated Facility)	OTC
Calendula Toothpaste Natural oral protection peppermint-free fluoride-free (Cleans and freshens the teeth and mouth, stimulates vascular development,aids slow-healing mucosa.)	WELEDA (Switzerland), made for USA distribution by Weleda Inc., Palisades, NY, 1-800-241-1030, http://usa.weleda.com	OTC
Oral Comfort All Natural Whitening Gel Toothpaste for Sensitive Teeth (Soothes sensitive teeth and gums; contains coenzyme Q_{10} for periodontal support.)	Jason Natural Cosmetics, Culver City, CA, 1-877-JASON-01, www.jason-natural.com	OTC
Echinacea Fresh Fluid Extract (Absorbed sublingually; inhibits viral reproduction and enhances WBC phagocytosis of bacteria via interferon-like activity facilitating healing of lesions.)	Scientific Botanicals, Seattle,WA, 1-206-527-5521, Available to physicians only	OTC

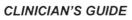
TABLE 12 – 1: COMPLEMETARY AND ALTERNATIVE DRUGS AND SUPPLEMENTS (CONTINUED)

Category / Product Name / Uses	Manufacturer / Contact Informtation	OTC / Rx
Lip Care		
Cold Sores Begone Topical Gel Robin (Treatment of cold sores; works best if applied according to directions when the first prodromal signs are experienced.)	Barr Enterprises, Inc., Mission Viejo, CA, 1-888-877-6315, www.csbegone.com	OTC
Cold Sore Relief (formerly Herpilyn Cream) (Relieves dryness, softens cold sores, fever blisters, and scabs.)	Lomapharm (Germany) for exclusive distribution by Enzymatic Therapy, Green Bay, WI, 1-800-783-2286	OTC
Unpetroleum SPF 18 Natural Lip Balm—vanilla, cherry, tangerine & wintermint (Soothes, protects, moisturizes, repairs.)	Avalon Natural Products, Twin Lakes, WI, 1-877-263-9456, wwwavalonnaturalproducts.com	OTC
Lip Rescue with Shea Butter Lip Balm (Apply to moisturize, heal or prevent dry, chapped lips.)	Desert Essence, Valencia, CA, 1-800-949-7331, www.desertessence.com	OTC
Burt's Bees Lifeguard's Choice Lip Balm Tube (Weatherproof lips from the drying effects of sun, wind and sea; 95% natural ingredients; also available as Fruit Flavored Lip Gloss & Beeswax Lip Balm.)	Burt's Bees, Inc., Durham, NC, 1-800-849-7112	OTC

OTC/RX = over-the-counter/prescription; WBC= white blood cell.

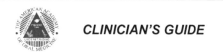
13 – MEDICATIONS FOR THE TREATMENT OF DRY MOUTH

Salivary gland hypofunction (SGH), or dry mouth, is a common condition that can cause significant oral discomfort and dysfunction leading to a number of complications. Xerostomia, which refers specifically to the patient's subjective report of oral dryness, may or may not reflect actual quantitative and/or qualitative salivary gland changes. In routine clinical use these terms are often used interchangeably. The most common causes of SGH are medications (eg, antihypertensive agents, antihistamines, diuretics, antidepressants, antipsychotics, and many others), autoimmune diseases (e.g., Sjögren syndrome, systemic lupus erythematosus, progressive systemic sclerosis, and chronic graft-versus-host disease), head and neck radiation involving the salivary glands (especially above 50 Gy), and dehydration. Regardless of the underlying cause, SGH is characterized by a marked decrease in salivary output, often accompanied by alterations in composition and consistency (thick, ropey, sticky), and notable dryness of the lips, oral mucosa and oropharynx (Figure 13-1). Although salivary flow rates (sialometry) and composition (sialochemistry) may be measured for research purposes, SGH is usually diagnosed based on a patient's subjective complaints of xerostomia along with objective visual clinical findings.

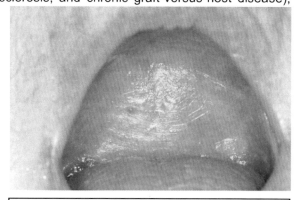

FIGURE 13-1
Dessicated and atrophic appearing palatal mucosa and tongue dorsum in a patient previously treated with radiation therapy for head and neck cancer.

Saliva is essential for its buffering and antimicrobial properties, remineralizing enamel, protecting the oral mucosa from trauma, chewing and swallowing foods, taste perception, and speech and communication. Without adequate salivary output, significant complications arise that may severely affect a patient's health and quality of life. Patients that have difficulty eating and swallowing may be at risk for malnutrition. Patients with little or no saliva frequently develop rampant caries, especially on the cervical and root surfaces (Figure 13-2). A dry mouth also increases the risk of developing oral candidosis, which causes further discomfort; patients with burning symptoms, mucosal erythema, or clinical signs of pseudomembranous candidosis (Figure 13-3) should be treated with appropriate antifungal therapy and followed closely long-term prophylaxis is often required. A dry mouth can also exacerbate existing periodontal disease.

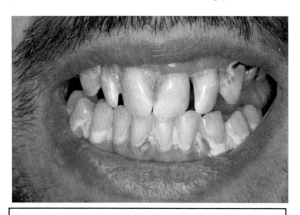

FIGURE 13-2
Rampant cervical and interproximal dental caries in a patient with chronic graft-versushost disease affecting the salivary glands. Note lichenoid mucosal changes of the labial mucosa as well.

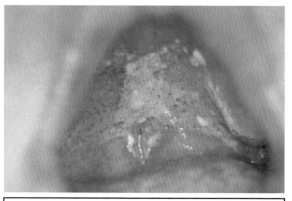

Figure 13-2
Pseudomembranous candidosis of the palate in a pateint previously treated with irradiation therapy.

When applicable, diagnosis, treatment, and/or management of any underlying etiology should be considered (Table 13-1). The signs and symptoms of xerostomia can be managed several ways. First, patients should be instructed to avoid caffeinated and alcoholic beverages, as these are extremely dehydrating. They should be encouraged to drink as much water as they comfortably can. The patient may carry a water bottle for frequent sipping; the direct lubricating effect can be quite helpful. Second, oral moisturizing agents and saliva substitutes offer various palliative options; patients may need to try several to find one they like. Third, for those patients that show some clinical evidence of residual functioning glands, sugarless (noncariogenic) gums and candies can effectively stimulate salivary flow. And fourth, systemic medications (sialogogues, muscarinic cholinergic agonists) that actually stimulate and increase salivary secretions may be prescribed. These may produce side effects that include excessive sweating and gastrointestinal upset; however most tolerate with few if any complications.

Patients should also be given a prescription for home fluoride treatments for prevention of dental caries (see Anticaries Section of Monograph), and see their dentist at least twice annually for regular care. Excellent home care is essential. Some patients may find that ordinary adult toothpastes cause intoloerable burning. In such cases, they should be advised to use a children's toothpaste or a specially formulated toothpaste such as Biotene (Table 13-1). Representative products and medications used to treat dry mouth are listed in Table 13-1.

TABLE 13 – 1: PHARMACEUTICALS FOR TREATMENT OF DRY MOUTH

Products	Manufacturer	OTC / Rx
Saliva Substitutes and Moisturizing Agents (representative products)		
Biotene Dry Mouth Toothpaste	GlaxoSmithKline, Philadelphia, PA	OTC
Biotene Gentle OTC, Mouthwash	GlaxoSmithKline, Philadelphia, PA	OTC, as needed
Moi-Stir	Kingswood Labs, Indianapolis, IN	OTC, as needed
Mouthkote	Parnell Pharmaceuticals, Inc., San Rafael, CA	OTC, as needed
OptiMoist Oral Moisturizer	Colgate-Palmolive Co., New York, NY	OTC, as needed
Oral Balance Liquid and Gel	Laclede, Inc., Rancho Domiguez, CA	OTC, as needed
Saliva Substitute	Roxane Laboratories, Ridgefield, CT	OTC, as needed
Salivart	Gebauer Company, Cleveland, OH	OTC, as needed
Thayer's Dry Mouth Lozenges	Henry Thayer Company,Westport, CT	OTC, as needed
Oasis Moisturizing Mouthwash and Mouth Spray	Gebauer Consumer Health Care, Cleveland, OH	OTC, as needed
MED Oral Dry Mouth Treatment	BHM Laboratories, Port Richey, FL	OTC, as needed
Saliva Stimulants		
Biotene Dry Mouth Gum	GlaxoSmithKline, Philadelphia, PA	OTC, as needed
Sugar-free candies/gums	Various	OTC, as needed
Pilocarpine hydrochloride (Salagen)	MGI Pharma Inc., Bloomington, MN	Rx, begin 5 mg three times a day, response may take 6–8 weeks
Cevimeline hydrochloride (Evoxac)	Daiichi Pharmaceutical Corp., Montvale, NJ	Rx, begin 30 mg three times a day, response time similar to pilocarpine HCL
Noncariogenic Sugar Substitutes		
Xylosweet sweetener, Spry gum and mints (xylitol)	Xlear, Inc., Orem, UT	OTC
TheraGum (xylitol)	Omni Pharmaceuticals	OTC

OTC/RX = over-the-counter/prescription

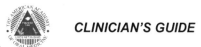

14 – OROFACIAL REACTIONS TO MEDICATIONS

The number of patients taking medications is continuously increasing, with an ever-growing number of individuals taking multiple pharmaceutical agents to manage one or more medical conditions. The increased use of medications is the result of the aging of the population and the fact that medications are now available to treat conditions that could not previously be managed with drugs. Drugs can have an impact on the oral mucosa or functions of the orofacial complex that the dentist is uniquely equipped to identify. Unfortunately, these manifestations can take a wide range of forms; none of which are absolutely unique to drug reactions, and all of which can be associated with other phenomena.

Adverse drug reactions is an all-inclusive term (Table 14-1) that includes side effects, which are undesirable drug effects that are secondary to the intended function or mechanism of the therapeutic agent. For example, scopolamine is a well-known anticholinergic agent used for the treatment of motion sickness. It also produces a dry mouth in two-thirds of patients—an expected but undesired result of the drug's antagonism of muscarinic receptors. Another example is long-term corticosteroids used to treat autoimmune diseases. The therapeutic immunosuppression caused by these drugs also predisposes the patient to opportunistic infections, including candidosis of the oral mucosa.

Another adverse drug reaction is an idiopathic reaction. As the term implies, these reactions are unexpected and unpredictable. These can be immunemediated conditions such as oral lichen planus–like lesions associated with thiazide diuretics.With others, such as dysgeusia and bruxism, the precise mechanism of the reaction is unclear.

EVALUATION OF SUSPECTED DRUG-RELATED ORAL REACTIONS

If you are concerned that an oral finding or complaint is related to a medication the patient is taking, there are several factors to consider.

1. Is the undesired reaction one that has been associated with a drug the patient is taking?
2. Did the undesired reaction start at the time when the drug therapy was initiated? (But keep in mind that drug reaction can take months to manifest)
3. Is the undesired oral reaction severe enough to merit a change in the patient's drug therapy?
4. Does discontinuing the drug eliminate the problem?

TREATMENT OF DRUG-RELATED ORAL REACTIONS

There are three options for treatment, depending on the problem and the patient's desires.

- The oral reaction can be attributed to the drug, but no intervention is necessary.
- The oral reaction is severe enough to merit treatment, but this can be accomplished locally without affecting the drug. For example, topical steroid therapy for drug-induced ulcerations.
- The oral reaction is severe enough to warrant discontinuing the patient's drug or switching to another drug with a similar therapeutic effect.

If the medication in question is prescribed by a physician, the physician should be the individual to discontinue or change the medication ut keep in mind that drug reactions can take months to manifest.)

TABLE 14 – 1: DRUG REACTIONS AND AGENTS COMMONLY RESPONSIBLE		
Drug Reaction	*Common Agents*	*Notes*
Lichenoid reactions	ACE inhibitors, beta blockers, NSAIDs (including COX-2 inhibitors), diuretics (especially thiazides), sulfonamides, dentifrices with cinnamonaldehyde, sulfamethoxazole, gold, hydroxychloroquine, allopurinol, lithium	Although reactions are often the reticular form of lichen planus, ulcerative and erosive lesions can also be observed.

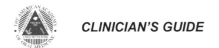
TABLE 14 – 1: DRUG REACTIONS AND AGENTS COMMONLY RESPONSIBLE (CONTINUED)

Drug Reaction	Common Agents	Notes
Aphthous-like ulcerations	NSAIDs, beta blockers, ACE inhibitors, protease inhibitors, nicorandil, methotrexate, cinnamonaldehyde, interferons, carbemazepine	Aphthous ulcerations are a common reaction and can come from any medicine.
Petechiae or hemorrhage	NSAIDs, warfarin, Coumadin, clopidogrel (Plavix)	
Blistering/erosions	Penicillamine, sulfasalazine, furosemide, NSAIDs, amoxicillin, vancomycin	
Bruxism and psychomotor symptoms	SSRIs, SNRIs	Some studies have shown an increase in nocturnal bruxism in young patients taking these drugs.
Xerostomia	Alcohol, antidepressants (SSRIs, SNRIs, TCAs, lithium, MAOIs), antipsychotics, benzodiazepines, antihistamines, anticholinergics, appetite suppressants, anti-acid production (H_2 blockers, PPIs), opiates, antihypertensives (α_2 agonists, beta blockers, diuretics), pseudoephedrine	Xerostomia is a subjective complaint. These manifestations may or may not coincide with clinically relevant reduction in saliva production.
Candidosis	Prednisone, cyclosporine, azathioprine, methotrexate, antibiotics	
Gingival enlargement	Calcium-channel blockers (nifedipine, verapamil), cyclosporine, phenytoin, (Dilantin), sodium valproate (Depakote), carbamezapine (Tegretol)	
Dysgeusia	ACE inhibitors, antifungals, carbemazepine, lithium, antithyroid medications (methimazole, methythiouracil, propothiouracil), antibiotics (especially β-lactams)	
Pigmentation changes	Tetracycline family drugs (both mucosa and teeth) (tetracycline and minocycline), oral contraceptives, hydroxychloroquine, chlorhexidine (extrinsic staining)	Tetracyclines can cause discolorations of teeth, but only in the developing dentition. Once permanent teeth are formed, there is no effect on the dentition.
Osteochemonecrosis	Alendronate (fosamax), pamindronate (Aredia), zolendronic acid (Zometa)	See Chapter 19 on bisphosphonates

ACE = angiotensin-converting enzyme; COX-2 = cyclooxygenase 2 inhibitor; MAOI = monoamine oxidase inhibitor; NSAID = nonsteroidal anti-inflammatory drug; PPI = protein pump inhibitor; SNRI = selective serotonin/norepinephrine reuptake inhibitor; SSRI = selective serotonin reuptake inhibitor; TCA = tricyclic antidepressant

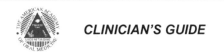

15 – THE HEMATOLOGIC IMPACT OF PHARMACOLOGY

A wide variety of pharmacologic agents may affect the patient's hematologic status; thus emphasizing the need for the clinician to have access to a contemporary reference resource. The basic laboratory studies used to evaluate the patient's hematologic status are the complete blood count with differential (CBCD) and tests of hemostasis: prothrombin time (PT), activated partial thromboplastin time (aPTT), and thrombin time (TT). The platelet function analyzer (PFA 100) is used to assess the adequacy of platelet function and has largely replaced the less accurate bleeding time test.

In assessing the potential affect of a medication on the patient's hematologic status, there are two major scenarios for which the clinician must have a basic understanding and appreciation. First, the dental patient may present for care with observable manifestations of a drug-induced blood dyscrasia (eg, fatigue in a patient taking dapsone or ecchymosis in an individual taking carbamazepine). Table 15-1 summarizes the signs and symptoms of the more common blood dyscrasias along with a partial listing of some of the more commonly implicated medications. The goal for the clinician is to recognize the signs and symptoms of a potential hematologic disorder and arrange for appropriate medical referral and management prior to delivering routine dental care.

In the second scenario, the dental patient may be on medication intended to target a component of the hematologic system (eg, daily acetylsalicylic acid [ASA] therapy to reduce platelet aggregation as a stroke preventive, or daily Coumadin therapy to reduce thromboembolic risk associated with a deep vein thrombophlebitis). Here, the goal for the clinician is to assess the patient's current overall health status and incorporate the necessary treatment modifications to render safe and appropriate dental care. Table 15-2 summarizes the management of such patients. As a rule, only the physician should modify any medically prescribed antiplatelet or anticoagulant regimen. For all surgical procedures, the technique should be as atraumatic as possible and local hemostatic measures, such as the use of primary closure and/or pressure packs should be utilized. The use of gelfoam/thrombin (or Oxycel, Surgicel, or microfibrillar collagen) and tranexamic acid may also be beneficial in stabilizing the clot. The use of supplemental pharmacological agents to control hemorrhage, such as desmopressin(DDAVP) and tranexamic acid (Cyklokapron), is rarely necessary and if undertaken should be coordinated by the patient's physician.

TABLE 15 – 1: SIGNS AND SYMPTOMS OF BLOOD DYSCRAISIAS AND COMMONLY IMPLICATED DRUGS		
Disorder	**Signs and Symptoms**	**Examples of Possible Causes**
Anemia	Pallor, fatigue, weakness, rapid pulse, shortness of breath, glossodynia, atrophic tongue	Antibiotics (dapsone, cephalosporins, rifampin), antihypertensives (hydrochlorothiazide, methyldopa), antimalarials (hydroxychloroquine, primaquine), antineoplastic agents (doxorubicin, etoposide), immunosuppressive agents (azathioprine, cyclosporine, gold salts, tacrolimus)
Aplastic anemia	Pallor, fatigue, weakness, rapid pulse, shortness of breath, petechiae, ecchymoses, purpura, abnormal gingival hemorrhage, epistaxis, infection	Antibiotics (chloramphenicol, sulfamethoxazole and trimethoprim), antineoplastic agents (asparaginase, cyclophosphamide, fluorouracil), phenothiazines (chlorpromazine, trifluoperazine), sulfonylureas (glyburide, tolbutamide)
Lymphopenia	Increased infection (particularly viral and fungal)	Antibiotics (ceftriaxone), antineoplastic agents (capecitabine, letrozole), imunosuppressive agents (muronomabe-CD3, thalidomide), interferons (interferon β-1b, peginterferon α-2a), monoclonal antibodies (alefacept, rituximab)

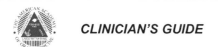

TABLE 15 – 1: SIGNS AND SYMPTOMS OF BLOOD DYSCRAISIAS AND COMMONLY IMPLICATED DRUGS (CONTINUED)

Disorder	Signs and Symptoms	Examples of Possible Causes
Neutropenia	Fever, infections such as cutaneous cellulitis, liver abscesses, furunculosis, pneumonia, and septicemia, stomatitis, gingivitis, perirectal inflammation, colitis, sinusitis, and otitis media often occur	ACE inhibitors (benazepril, captopril, lisinopril), analgesics (acetaminophen, ibuprofen, sulindac), antibiotics (chloramphenicol, cephalosporins), antineoplastic agents (asparaginase, fluorouracil, methotrexate, rituximab), antirheumatic drugs (gold salts, etanercept)
Thrombocytopenia	Petechiae, ecchymoses, purpura, spontaneous or prolonged gingival hemorrhage, epistaxis	Antiarrhythmic agents (disopyramide, sulfamethoxazole and trimethoprim), anticonvulsant agents (carbamazepine, valproic acid), antineoplastic agents (asparaginase, cyclophosphamide, fluorouracil, methotrexate, rituximab), immunosuppressive agents (azathioprine, cyclosporine), interferons (interferon β-1b, peginterferon α-2a), sulfonylureas (glyburide, tolbutamide)
Thrombocytopathy	Petechiae, ecchymoses, purpura, spontaneous or prolonged gingival hemorrhage, epistaxis	NSAIDs (aspirin, ibuprofen, diflunisal), antiplatelet agents (clopidogrel, ticlopidine)
Coagulopathy	Petechiae, ecchymoses, purpura, hemarthrosis, delayed hemorrhage, epistaxis	Anticoagulants (dalteparin, enoxaparin, heparin, warfarin)

TABLE 15 – 2: MANAGEMENT GUIDELINES FOR PATIENTS WITH POTENTIAL HEMOSTATIC IMPAIRMENT

Scenario	Management Guidelines
Patient on ASA or NSAID therapy for routine pain control (ASA, ibuprofen)	Generally no dosage adjustment necessary for routine dental care including minor surgery. If more extensive surgery is necessary, advise patient to discontinue medication to allow for adequate platelet replenishment. • For ASA: discontinue for 3–5 days • For other NSAIDs: discontinue for 2 days
Patient on prescribed antiplatelet therapy (ASA, ASA and dipyridamole, cilostazol, clopidogrel, ticlopidine)	Generally no dosage adjustment necessary or recommended for routine dental care including minor surgery. For more extensive surgery, a medical consultation is warranted • Physician may direct patient to discontinue antiplatelet therapy as described above, typically for 5-7 days. • Physician may prescribe additional steps to be used such as the presurgical administration of DDAVP
Outpatient on prescribed anticoagulant therapy (warfarin)	Verify INR on day of treatment. • If INR < 3.5, okay for dental care • If INR > 3.5, consult with physician warranted. Only the physician should prescribe any necessary dosage adjustments in anticoagulant therapy.

ASA = acetylsalic acid; INR = international normalized ratio; NSAID = nonsteroidal anti-inflammatory drug.

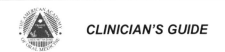
16 – EXTEMPORANEOUSLY COMPOUNDED AGENTS FOR DENTAL USE

Extemporaneously compounded drug products are formulated and produced by pharmacists and prescribed by practitioners to meet patient-specific pharmacotherapeutic needs. These preparations consist of US Food and Drug Administration (FDA)–approved drugs prepared in specialized delivery vehicles or in combinations for specific management of oral and facial conditions.

Most compounded products prescribed by oral medicine clinicians are designed for topical and/or local use on the skin or mucosa to affect surface pathosis or to penetrate to subepithelial tissue abnormalities. These agents are often prescribed when patients have not adequately responded to mainstream, mass-marketed prescription drug products. The intent of compounded formulations is to supplant or supplement the pharmacotherapeutic benefit of systemically prescribed drugs, thereby minimizing adverse effects and maximizing therapeutic efficacy.

The purpose of compounded medications is to fill a void in the pharmacotherapeutic arsenal available to health-care practitioners. It is neither appropriate, nor legal, for pharmacists to copy commercially available products or to supply compounded products to practitioners which are sold to the patient from an office setting.

The extemporaneous compounding of pharmaceutical products is best undertaken by pharmacists with experience and specific training in the area. These "compounding pharmacists" often belong to one or more associations that specialize in disseminating information regarding the stability and efficacy of a wide variety of formulations. While compounded medications have benefited many patients, it is important to remember that these formulations have not undergone the in vivo efficacy and safety studies that drug companies are required to submit prior to releasing a product to the market.

Dental practitioners request, for example, combinations of products such as dentifrices with added antimicrobial agents, fluoride-chlorhexidine combinations, stannous fluoride products, or triamcinolone rinses in saline vehicles, which are not appropriate because of specific incompatibility issues. A frequent request of compounding pharmacists is to make the product more palatable for the patient by adding such agents as sweeteners or flavorings. In the case of chlorhexidine, for example, many flavors and sweetening agents will inactivate the drug.

Practitioners trained in the scientific method often have difficulty accepting novel formulations when there is little or no primary literature available on the product. Many anecdotal "miracle cures" have failed the test of controlled clinical trials. Requests for products no longer on the market should only be made once it has been established that the product was not withdrawn for safety or efficacy issues.

Table 16-1 contains examples of extemporaneously compounded products that have been used by dental practitioners and specialists in the mitigation of a variety of oral and facial conditions. It is our intent to increase the awareness of our dental colleagues about these agents for the benefit of them and their patients.

Note: If you, as a practitioner feel you need a specifically compounded product, please contact a compounding pharmacist to see if it can be created. Examples of these pharmacists are given below.

Clinical Specialties
3708 Executive Center Drive
Augusta, GA 30907

Health Dimensions Compounding Pharmacy
39303 Country Club Drive A-26
Farmington Hills, MI 48331

Custom Prescription Shoppe at DuraMed
1543 15th Street
Augusta, GA 30901

Nucara Pharmacy
1150 Fifth Street
City Center Square
Coralville IA 52241

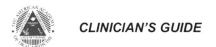
TABLE 16– 2: EXAMPLES OF EXTEMPORANEOUSLY COMPOUNDED PRODUCTS

Indications & Compounds	Information
Antifungal	
• Amphotericin B oral rinse or troches	Amphotericin oral rinse was discontinued by the manufacturer due to lack of sales.
• Nystatin rinse (sugar-free)	Commercially available nystatin rinses contain 30–50% sucrose.
• Clotrimazole troches	
Burning Mouth or Mucositis	
• Clonazepam oral troches	Troches are designed for slow release of medication in the oral cavity. They provide topical and usually systemic effects.
• Amitriptyline oral troches	
Myofascial Pain (extraoral)	
• Ketoprofen, cyclobenzaprine, carbamazepine or gabapentin in PLO gel	PLO gel is a common vehicle used for transdermal delivery of anti-inflammatory agents and analgesics. Works well on trigger points.
Neuralgic Pain (extraoral)	
• Guaifenisin, dextromethorphan, carbamazepine in speed gel	Speed gel is a variation of the PLO gel and provides fast onset.
• Ketoprofen, gabapentin, ketamine in PLO gel	
Oral Ulcerative Disease	
• Micronized triamcinolone acetonide 0.1 or 0.2% oral rinse	Triamcinolone rinse is unflavored & used for 1 min up to qid (pc & hs), NPO 30 min after use and must be compounded with sterile water for irrigation.
• Fluocinonide or clobetasol in Orabase type vehicle	Provides more potent corticosteroid delivery than commercial triamcinolone in Orabase product.
• Misoprostol in mucoadhesive powder	Can be of use in lesions unresponsive to steroids.
Perioral Dermatitis	
• Ketoprofen, mupirocin, bacitracin	Apply thin film four times daily.

PLO gel = pluronic lecithin organgel.

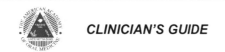
17 – PHARMACOLOGIC CONSIDERATION FOR TOBACCO CESSATION

Tobacco use has been identified as the chief avoidable cause of illness and death in the United States, being responsible for more than 440,000 deaths each year. It is estimated that 22.5% of the adult population smokes tobacco, and about 2,200 adolescents initiate smoking daily. The 1988 US Surgeon's Report established nicotine as the primary addictive agent in tobacco. When tobacco users attempt to quit, they will more than likely experience withdrawal symptoms as characterized in the Diagnostic and Statistical Manual ofMental Disorders (DSM) IV. These symptoms include dysphoric or depressed mood, insomnia, irritability, frustration, anger, difficulty concentrating, restlessness, decreased heart rate, and increased appetite or weight gain. Although nicotine does have a short halflife, withdrawal symptoms can last well beyond the initial phase of nicotine abstinence: from 48 hours (lightheadedness) to more than 10 weeks (increased appetite). The risk for relapse can extend beyond 1 year postcessation.

The current best practice approach for assisting the nicotine-dependent tobacco user combines behavior modification with pharmacotherapy (Table 17-1).

Nicotine Replacement Therapy (NRT). NRT is designed to provide relief from tobacco withdrawal by replacing sufficient levels of nicotine from an alternative source in the absence of other harmful substances in tobacco. Dose is generally reduced over time, or a period of approximately 3–6 months.

Bupropion SR (Wellbutrin SR, Zyban). Bupropion SR is the first non-nicotine product approved by the US Food and Drug Administration for the treatment of nicotine dependence. Its therapeutic affect is believed to derive from both dopaminergic and noradrenergic activity.

Varenicline (Chantix). Varenicline is another non-nicotine product approved by the US Food and Drug Administration for the treatment of nicotine dependence. Its therapeutic effect is achieved by partially agonizing nicotine receptors, thus reducing craving and withdrawal. It also antagonizes nicotine at the same site which reduces pleasure associated with tobacco use.

TABLE 17 - 1: DRUGS OF CHOICE FOR USE IN TOBACCO CESSATION

Medication 1st Line Options	Proper Use	Advantages	Disadvantages
Nicotine Transdermal Patch (Nicoderm, Nicotrol, Habitrol)	Stop tobacco 1 per day, on awakening 9–12 weeks Tapering option	Effective blood levels within 1–2 hours Simple to use; 3 dose levels No new drug; Eliminates "tar"and CO Concern re: use with tobacco overstated	Skin-related side effects common Caution with CV disease Max dose may not be enough for some
Nicotine Polacrilex ('gum') (Nicorette)	Stop tobacco Chew minimally and park for 30 minutes 1 piece every 1–2 hours Up to 24 pieces per day 12 weeks	2 mg (up to 24 cigarettes per day) 4 mg (25 or more cigarettes per day) Orange / Mint / Regular Oral substitute; Use as needed Good for "irregular" smoker	Insufficient use is common Chewing too much increases side effects Taste can be Unpleasant (original flavor) No food or drink before or while using

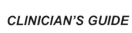
TABLE 17 - 1: DRUGS OF CHOICE FOR USE IN TOBACCO CESSATION (CONTINUED)			
Medication 1st Line Options	**Proper Use**	**Advantages**	**Disadvantages**
Nicotine Inhaler (Nicotrol)	Stop tobacco 6–16 cartridges per day 12 weeks; can taper over 1–12 additional weeks Stop if not quit in 4 weeks	Easy to tailor Oral substitute	Lower level of delivery—may not be ideal for heavier users as sole therapy Costly
Nicotine Nasal Spray (Nicotrol NS)	Stop tobacco 1–2 doses per hour (1 dose = 1 spray in each nostril) Max: 5 doses per hour (40 doses/ day) Do not inhale while spraying 12 weeks Stop if not quit in 4 weeks	May be more useful with heavier users	Irritation of nasal tract Cost
Nicotine Lozenge (Commit)	Stop tobacco Absorbed via oral mucosal No eating or drinking 15 minutes before use Up to 6 per 5-hour period, max of 20 per day 12 weeks	2 mg (1st cigarette after 30 min of awakening) 4 mg (1st cigarette sooner than 30 min) Oral substitute Use as needed Good for "irregular" smoker	Consuming to fast can cause side effects No food or drink before or while using
Bupropion SR (Zyban)	Once per day for 3 days, then twice per day for at least 7–12 weeks (up to 6 months) Tapering at end of treatment not necessary	Ease of use Can initiate while still using tobacco Antidepressant effect	h/o seizure or eating disorder Abrupt stopping of alcohol, sedatives No MAOI or other form of Bupropion 1–2 weeks to reach adequate blood levels
Varenicline (Chantix)	0.5 mg per day for 3 days, then 0.5 mg twice per day for 4 days, then 1 mg twice per day for 11 weeks If quit at 12 weeks, consider another 12 weeks Starter Pak and Continuation Pak Eat and full glass of water	Best outcomes to date No CYP450 (liver) concerns No drug-drug interactions	Nausea Should not be combined with NRT

COPD = chronic obstructive pulmonary disease; CV = cardiovascular disease; MAOI = monoamine oxidase inhibitor; NRT = nicotine replacement therapy.

Prescribing medications will produce a reliable increase in quit rates; however, incorporation of a brief counseling-based component will significantly increase the percentage of successful quitters over the self-quit rate, yielding 12 to 15% at 1 year.

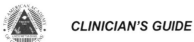
The Public Health Service Guideline, Treating Tobacco Use and Dependence (2000), provides evidence-based recommendations regarding clinical and systems interventions that will increase the likelihood of successful quitting. Every oral health care provider who treats tobacco-dependent patients should be familiar with the contents of this manual. Several important issues are raised, such as the positive linear relationship between treatment time (in minutes or sessions) and success rate, as well as effective treatment components (eg, problem solving, social support). In addition, the Guideline describes the well-researched 5A model of intervention with tobacco users. This model ensures that every patient is Asked about their tobacco use, Advised to quit, Assessed for readiness to quit, Assisted if ready to quit by setting a quit date, receiving motivational literature and pharmacotherapy, and Arranged for follow-up care. These interventions are designed to take 3 min or less per visit, divided among members of the healthcare team. This level of intervention should be the minimal level of service offered to any tobacco user who desires to quit.

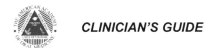

18 – ELECTRONIC AND PDA RESOURCES IN PHARMACOLOGY

One of the most critical aspects of the medical history remains a comprehensive list of all medications, herbal preparations, and nutraceuticals the patient is using. It is important that this list include dosages and frequency of use with as much detail as possible. Although significant as a record, the real task is to interpret the medication list. One must thus determine, for example, if the drugs pose any contraindications to treatment, require any laboratory testing, or create any additional considerations with respect to drugs the dentist may prescribe.

The real challenge arises in the fact that pharmaceuticals are an ever-changing arena. New drugs are constantly arriving on the market, drugs are being removed from the market, new dosages and extended-release forms become available, and new interactions and side effects are recognized. Furthermore, the same active ingredient may carry innumerable different trade names that are not remotely similar in appearance! It is both unreasonable and impossible for any clinician to remain completely current with all of these changes and have a flawless working knowledge of all commercially available pharmaceuticals. Regardless, dental professionals still remain responsible for the safe and appropriate treatment of their patients. Fortunately, the digital age offers many solutions to these problems.

Evaluation of the medications and determining their US Food and Drug Administration (FDA)-approved indications for disease treatment requires the use of appropriate reference materials. Traditional methods would include use of a drug index textbook such as the *Physician's Desk Reference* (PDR) or American Society of Health-System Pharmacists AHFS Drug Information books. Although helpful, problems with the timeliness of the information contained within these texts can occur, as they are typically released on an annual basis.

Electronic forms of full-text drug databases are readily available and user friendly. These databases are updated regularly and this obviates the problem of containing out-of-date information. These databases include Internet-accessed databases such as *AHFS Drug Information, Clinical Pharmacology, Clinical Reference Library, DRUGDEX Information Systems, Drug Facts and Comparisons,* and the *Physician's Desk Reference* (PDR). These are available online and have user-friendly interfaces. Information can also be printed for future reference or for distribution to patients.

Personal digital assistant (PDA)-based applications are also a popular means of obtaining information on many topics including drugs. PDA are readily available and widely used by almost all members of society. More recently smart phones (mobiles phones with advanced functionality and computer like interface) are being used by healthcare professionals in obtaining drug database information. There are many options available to the PDA and smart phone user wishing to obtain drug information. These options include the widely used applications such ePocrates, LexiDrug, and Pocket PDR. The advantage to this is that the clinician can literally carry the reference on their person at all times. Many of these references also allow the clinician to check for drug interactions by entering multiple drugs, contain information about drug prices, or contain formulary information (Table 18-1).

As needs differ between practitioners, one should evaluate these programs prior to purchasing. One should consider ease of use, completeness and accuracy of information, frequency of updates, memory requirements, and cost. Some applications are free and others require subscriptions or annual fees. Table 18-1 is not meant to be exhaustive, and is intended as a general guide to the various software systems available for PDA /smart phone drug information systems.

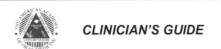

TABLE 18 - 1: ELECTRONIC RESOURCES FOR DRUG INFORMATION

Reference Source	Web Site
Web Resource for Pharmacology (free)	
Medline Plus Drug Information	www.nlm.nih.gov/medlineplus/druginformation.html
	Searchable drug database by name for thousands of prescription and OTC drugs.
MedicineNet.com	www.medicinenet.com/medications/article.htm
	Searchable drug database by name for thousands of prescription and OTC drugs. Contains good information but more geared toward patients.
PDR.net	www.pdr.net
	Excellent and comprehensive resource that contains all information in the print PDR as well as up-to-date resources about new drug approvals and warnings. Resources are also available to provide to patients. Updates at regular intervals.
PDA/Smart Phone Resources Available by Fee or Subscription	
AHFS Drug source	http://www.skyscape.com/estore/ProductDetail.aspx?ProductId=1188
DrDrugs	http://www.skyscape.com/estore/productdetail.aspx?productid=220
A 2 Z Drugs	http://www.skyscape.com/EStore/ProductDetail.aspx?ProductID=218
ePocrates Rx Pro	www.lexi.com
DrugDex	http://www.micromedex.com/products/drugdex/
Medical Wizards Davis's Drug Guide (PDA Only)	http://www.medicalwizards.com/products/view/id/84
PDA/Smart Phone Resources Available at No cost	
ePocrates	www.ePocrates.com
Pocket PDR (PDA only)	http://www.pdr.net/home/pdrhome.aspx

PDA = personal digital assistant; PDR = Physician's Desk Reference; OTC = over-the-counter.

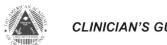

19 – BISPHOSPHONATES

The chemicals known as bisphosphonates have been known since the midnineteenth century. They were not used as biologically active compounds for drug therapy until the 1970s. Bisphosphonates are synthetic analogs of inorganic pyrophosphate that have a high affinity for calcium. They are rapidly cleared from the circulation, and bind to bone mineral, selectively concentrating in bone. The drug not incorporated in bone is not metabolized and is eliminated in urine. Bisphosphonates are potent inhibitors of osteoclast activity and slow bone resorption. The drug incorporated into the mineralized bone matrix accumulates over extended periods of time and may take years to be completely eliminated. During bone resorption bisphosphonates are released from the bone surface and may be reincorporated into newly formed bone or internalized into osteoclasts. The latter process results in loss of the ability of osteoclasts to resorb bone and promote apoptosis.

There are several different indications for drugs of the bisphosphonate class. They are used to treat hypercalcemia of malignancy, bone metastases of various types of cancer like breast, lung, prostate, and multiple myeloma, and osteoporosis. These medications are available for delivery via the oral and intravenous (IV) routes, and the decision on what bisphosphonate to use is dependent on the type of condition being treated and the potency of the drug. Recently, a formulation of bisphosphonates has become available that is administered as a single yearly IV infusion. This potency is also directly related to the nitrogen content of the bisphosphonate and the complexity of the nitrogen-containing "R" group.

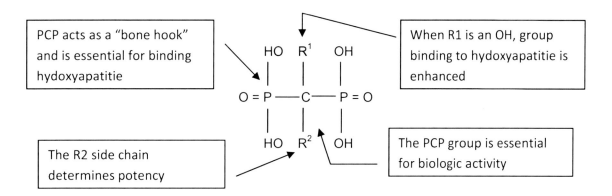

FIGURE 19-1. Chemical structure of bisphosphonates demonstrating how the manipulation of the basic structure will change the biological activity and the potency of the drug. (Licata AA. Discovery, clinical development, and therapeutic uses of bisphosphonates. Ann Pharmacother 2005;39:668–77)

TABLE 18 - 1: RELATIVE BISPHOSPHONATES POTENCIES	
Compound	*Preclinical Antiresorptive Relative Potency*
Short alkyl or halide side chain etidronate	1
Cyclic chloro side chaintiludronate	10
Aminoterminal group	
pamidronate	100
alendronate	100–1,000
Cyclic nitrogen-containing side chain	
risedronate	1,000–10,000
ibandronate	1,000–10,000
zoledronic acid	≥ 10,000

Treatment of osteoporosis with bisphosphonates. Endocrinol Metab Clin North Am 1998;27:419–39.

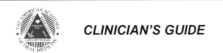

Recently, cases of osteonecrosis involving the maxilla and mandible have been reported to the literature in patients receiving bisphosphonate therapy. At the time of publication, there were hundreds of such cases reported between 2003 and 2007. Of these cases, over 94% occurred in patients being treated with IV formulations of zolendrenate and pamidronate. Cases have been reported in patients taking oral bisphosphonates (alendronate, risedronate, ibandronate, and clodronate) as well. The use of bisphosphonate seems to be the only common link in the cases reported, although other factors such as diabetes, corticosteroid use, and tobacco use may play a role.

TABLE 19 - 2: TABLE OF COMMERCIALLY AVAILABLE BISPHOSPHONATES			
Brand	*Generic*	*Administration*	*Indication*
Aredia	Pamidronate	IV infusion	Metastatic bone disease Hypercalcemia of malignancy
Zometa	Zoledronic acid	IV infusion	Metastatic bone disease Hypercalcemia of malignancy
Fosamax	Alendronate	Oral	Osteoporosis Osteopenia
Boniva	Ibandronate	IV / Oral	Osteoporosis
Actonel	Risedronate	Oral	Osteoporosis

Most cases of bisphosphonate-associated osteonecrosis have been observed after invasive dental procedures such as extraction, surgical periodontal procedures, and other trauma. However, some cases have been reported as occurring spontaneously and without any precipitating factors. The hallmark of this condition is a nonhealing area of exposed bone after several weeks of proper care. A generally accepted criterion for diagnosis is delayed or absent healing that lasts 6 or more weeks. Usually, the condition begins asymptomatically. As the exposed areas of bone become infected, the patient may begin to feel pain, and if the infection becomes severe in the mandible, the patient may experience paresthesia or numbness.

Treatment is difficult, as bisphosphonate-associated osteonecrosis does not respond well to most therapies, and aggressive intervention may even cause the condition to worsen and increase the area of involvement. There is no standardized treatment or accurate accounting of the efficacy of particular treatment modalities. The current thinking is that conservative treatment is best, including:

- Removal only of dead bone (ie, sequestra or involucra) without extension to adjacent normal tissues
- Minimal manipulation of soft tissue surrounding necrotic bone
- Antiseptic rinses such as chlorhexidine gluconate 0.12% three times daily
- Systemic antibiotic therapy such as amoxicillin or a penicillin family drug in combination with metronidazole

The exact mechanism that leads to the formation of osteonecrosis is unknown. Current thinking posits that bisphosphonates, by disrupting osteoclastic activity, impair the healing process after traumatic injury. Additionally, bisphosphonates are known to have antiangiogenic properties: reducing the growth of new blood vessels can also impair healing and likely plays a role in this process.

GUIDELINES FOR PREVENTION OF OSTEONECROSIS IN PATIENTS TAKING BISPHOSPHONATES

- Ideally, patients should receive a complete dental evaluation prior to initiation of bisphosphonate therapy.
- Potential sources of infection and trauma should be eliminated. Hopeless teeth must be extracted and prosthodontic appliances should be adjusted to prevent trauma.

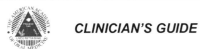
In a patient taking a bisphosphonate drug:

- If possible, endodontic therapy and retention of teeth is preferable to extraction.
- Invasive dental treatment including extractions, periodontal surgery, and placement of dental implants should be well-planned. Atraumatic technique must be used. Endodontic therapy with maintenance of the roots may be indicated over a tooth extraction.
- Patients should ***not*** be advised to stop taking bisphosphonates to avoid developing osteonecrosis. Because of the long half-life of these medications and the fact that they are slowly released from bone, there is no evidence that discontinuing the drug will reduce the risk of osteonecrosis.
- CTX testing. C-terminal telopeptide is a normal product of bone metabolism. Recently, some authors have devised a test for predicting the risk of osteonecrosis based on sequential measurements o f this protein. However, these results have not been validated or confirmed by multiple studies. At this time this test is not endorsed as the standard for risk assessment.

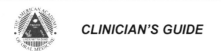

REFERENCES

American Dental Association Council on Scientific Affairs. Dental management of patients receiving oral bisphosphonate therapy: expert panel recommendations. J Am Dent Assoc 2006;137:1144–50.

American Dental Association, American Academy of Orthopaedic Surgeons. Antibiotic prophylaxis for dental patients with total joint replacements Advisory Statement. J Am Dent Assoc 2003; 134:895–9.

Brown RS, Rhodus NL. Epinephrine and local anesthesia revisited. Oral Surg Oral Med Oral Pathol Oral Radiol Endod 2005;100:401–8.

Brown RS, Rhodus NL.Epinephrine and local anesthesia revisited.

Cigarette smoking among adults—United States, 2006. MMWR 2007;56.

DeRossi S, Hersh EV. Antibiotics and oral contraceptives. Dent Clin N Am 2002;46:653–64.

Estilo CS, Van Poznak CH, Williams T, et al. Osteonecrosis of the maxilla and mandible in patients treated with bisphosphonates: a retrospective study. Proc Am Soc Clin Oncol 2004; 22:750, abs # 8088.

Fiore MC, Bailey WC, Cohen SJ, et al. Treating tobacco use and dependence. Clinical practice guideline. Rockville, MD: U.S. Department of Health and Human Services; Public Health Service. June 2000.

Fleisch H. Bisphosphonates in bone disease: From the laboratory to the patients. San Diego: Academic Press; 2000. p 34–5.

Gallo WJ, Ellis E. Efficacy of diphenhydramine hydrochloride for local anesthesia before oral surgery. J Am Dent Assoc Vol 115: 263–66 Oral Surg Oral Med Oral Pathol Oral Radiol Endod 2005;100(4):401–8.

Handbook of Local Anesthesia, Malamed SF, 5 ed,Mosby/Elsevier, 2004.

Jeske AH, Suchko GD. Lack of a scientific basis for routine discontinuation of oral anticoagulation therapy before dental treatment. J Am Dent Assoc 2003;134:1492–7.

Lacy CF, Armstrong LL, Goldman MP, Lance LL. Drug information handbook. 12th ed. Hudson, OH: Lexi-Comp; 2004.

Little JW, Falace DA, Miller CS, Rhodus NL. Bleeding disorders. In: Dental management of the medically compromised patient, ed 6. St. Louis: Mosby; 2002. p. 332–64.

Lockhart PB, Loven B, Brennan MT, Fox PC. The evidence base for the efficacy of antibiotic prophylaxis in dental practice. J Am Dent Assoc 2007;138:458–74.

Marx RE. Pamidronate (aredia) and zoledronate (zometa) induced avascular necrosis of the jaws: a growing epidemic. J Maxillofac Surg 2003;61:1115–8.

Migliorati CA, Casiglia J, Epstein J, et al. Managing the care of patients with bisphosphonateassociated osteonecrosis.An American Academy of Oral Medicine position paper. J Am Dent Assoc 2005;136:1658–68.

Migliorati CA. Bisphosphonates and oral cavity avascular necrosis of bone. J Clin Oncol 2003;21:4253–4.

Pindborg JJ. Classification of oral lesions associated with HIV infection. Oral Surg Oral Med Oral Pathol 1989; 67:292–5.

Rogers MJ,Watts DJ, Russel RGG.Overview of bisphosphonates. Cancer Suppl 1997; 80:1652–60.

Ruggiero SL,Mehrotra B,Rosenberg TJ, Engroff SL. Osteonecrosis of the jaws associated with the use of bisphosphonates: A review of 63 cases. J Oral Maxillofac Surg 2004;62:527–34.

Sato M, Grasser W, Endo N, et al. Bisphosphonate action. Alendronate localization in rat bone and effects on osteoblast ultrastructure. J Clin Invest 1991;88:2095–105.

Sietsema WK, Ebantino FH, Salvagno AM, Bevan JA. Antiresoptive dose-dependent relationship across three generations of bisphosphonates. Drugs Exp Clin Res 1989;15:389–96.

US Department of Health and Human Services. The Health consequences of smoking: nicotine addiction. A report of the Surgeon General. Atlanta (GA): US Department of Health and Human Serices. Public Halth Service, Centers for Disease Control, Center for Chronic Disease Prevention and Health Promotion. Office of Smoking and Health. DHHS Publication No. (PHS) (CDC).

Wilson W, Taubert KA, Gewitz M, et al. Prevention of Infective Endocarditis. Guidelines from the American Heart Association. A Guideline From the American Heart Association Rheumatic Fever, Endocarditis, and Kawasaki Disease Committee, Council on Cardiovascular Disease in the Young, and the Council on Clinical Cardiology, Council on Cardiovascular Surgery and Anesthesia, and the Quality of Care and Outcomes Research Interdisciplinary Working Group. Circulation 2007;116:1736-1754.

www.pfizerpro.com/brands/chantix.jsp (accessed December 2007).

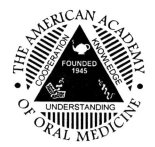

The American Academy of Oral Medicine
P.O. Box 2016
Edmonds, Washington 98020
Phone 425.778.6162   Fax 425.771.9588
www.aaom.com   Email: Info@aaom.com

Application for Membership

Nominations must be returned as soon as possible to be acted upon at the next Academy meeting.

Eligibility for Membership

1. Nominee for **Regular Membership** shall be a graduate of an accredited Dental School or Medicine School and shall be a member of his/her representative National Society and shall pursue special interest or accomplishment in the field of Oral Medicine.

2. Nominee for **Affiliate Membership** (student) shall be a graduate of an accredited Dental or Medical School and shall be a member of his/her representative National Society and currently in training in a Postdoctoral program.

3. This application form should be **accompanied by a check (U.S. Funds) for $295.00 for Active Membership or $145.00 for Affiliate Membership (student)** which includes the one-time initiation fee. In event membership is not acted upon favorably, the total fee will be refunded. Make all checks payable to The American Academy of Oral Medicine, Inc. (Foreign checks must be made payable in U.S. Funds through a U.S. Bank.) The fiscal year for dues starts January 1.

4. After acceptance into the Academy, Active Membership dues are $295.00 annually and Affiliate Membership (student) dues are $145.00 annually, which shall include a subscription to ORAL SURGERY, ORAL MEDICINE, ORAL PATHOLOGY, ORAL RADIOLOGY, and ENDODONTOLOGY.

Dues are payable prior to election.

5. **Please attach a copy of your curriculum vitae or resume and a recent photo, for publication purposes, with this application.**

Applicant Name _____ **Degree** _____

Office Address _____

Telephone _____   Fax _____

Home Address _____

Telephone _____   Fax _____

Preferred Mailing address _____ Office _____ Home   Date _____

Email address _____

Sponsor (Academy Member, Please Print) _____

Sponsor's Signature _____

Date _____

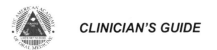
1. Predental Education _____
   College, dates, and degrees _____
2. Dental and Professional Postdoctoral Education _____
   Schools, dates, and degrees _____
3. Licensed to practice dentistry, date(s), location(s) _____
4. Types of specialty and years in specialty practice _____
5. Are you certified in that specialty? _____ If yes, date certified _____
6. Membership in professional societies _____
   _____
   _____

7. Government Service, Military or Civilian (at present, not reserve status)
   (a) Service _____   (b) Rank _____
8. Teaching service in dental, medical or other schools
   (a) Name of School _____
   (b) Title _____
   (c) Subject Taught _____ (d) Date _____
9. Hospital Staff or Services
   Staff Rank _____ Dates _____
10. Research in progress & completed (attach information) _____
    _____
    _____

11. Why are you interested in AAOM membership? _____
    _____

12. Has your license to practice in ANY state or jurisdiction been limited, suspended or revoked?
    _____No   _____Yes   If yes, please explain on attached sheet.
13. Has your DEA certificate to prescribe controlled substances been investigated, limited, suspended, revoked or restricted in any way or voluntarily or involuntarily been relinquished?
    _____No   _____Yes   If yes, please explain on attached sheet.
14. Have you privileges in ANY hospital been denied, suspended, reduced, revoked or not renewed or involuntarily been relinquished?
    _____No   _____Yes   If yes, please explain on attached sheet.
15. Have you had an adverse decision against you in a malpractice action and/or Federal tort claim?
    _____No   _____Yes   If yes, please explain on attached sheet.
16. Have you had any felony criminal convictions?
    _____No   _____Yes   If yes, please explain on attached sheet.

I attest that the statements in this application are true.

Applicant Signature _____

FOR OFFICE USE ONLY   Date of Election _____

Action considered by Board (Approved or Tabled)

_____   _____
Membership Chair   Date

Return application to AAOM, P.O. Box 2016, Edmonds, Washington 980202. Phone: 425.778.6162   REV 08.18.09

Made in United States
North Haven, CT
14 October 2022

25460342R00033